# Emergency Orthopedics

Sven-Anders Sölveborn

# Emergency Orthopedics

## A Manual on Acute Conditions of the Locomotor System

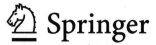 Springer

Sven-Anders Sölveborn
Hospital of Ystad
Ystad
Sweden

Translation of the Swedish language edition
Sölveborn: Ortopedi på akuten
© 2007 by Norstedts akademiska Förlag, Studentlitteratur
Illustrations by Ronnie Nilsson
This translation of the title is published by arrangement with Studentlitteratur AB, Sweden.

ISBN 978-3-642-41853-2    ISBN 978-3-642-41854-9 (eBook)
DOI 10.1007/978-3-642-41854-9
Springer Heidelberg New York Dordrecht London

Library of Congress Control Number: 2013958417

Printed on acid-free paper

Springer is part of Springer Science+Business Media (www.springer.com)

# Preface

*Emergency Orthopaedics* is a practical and comprehensive manual, describing how to diagnose and treat acute orthopaedic problems. The reader is offered assistance in identifying the injury/disorder and the author gives firm and up-to-date advice on the short term and long term aspects of treatment.

For every condition, the author has extracted such facts that could have practical importance for the management of the disorder. The book has a problem-based approach since the chapter headings consist of the main symptom that the patient presents.

The illustrations are extraordinarily instructive and include guidance on issues usually raised in the E.D., and that are often not included in other literature, such as practical manual measures like reductions (of fractures and joint dislocations) and examination techniques.

Sven-Anders Sölveborn is a senior orthopaedic officer with a very long experience of clinical work, research and education. The book is written with the wisdom that follows extensive practical experience of work in emergency rooms. The author is also an internationally recognized authority in sports medicine and the book offers extremely useful elements of sports medicine principles.

The book is a real treasure-trove, especially for internship doctors, specialty registrars (resident physicians), general practitioners, nurses and other staff in the emergency room. Physiotherapists, chiropractors, and naprapaths will also find the book useful. I warmly recommend it.

Linköping, Sweden

Jan Ekstrand
Chief physician in orthopaedics
and professor of Sports Medicine
University Hospital of Linköping

# About the Author

Specialist in orthopaedic surgery and certified sports medicine physician, senior officer and former head of the orthopaedic department, now director of internship education for the Hospital of Ystad, Sweden, former researcher at the Uppsala University, past-president of the Swedish Society of Sports Medicine, now Secretary-General of the North European Chapter of Sports & Exercise Medicine, physician to the Swedish national association of handball, well-known lecturer, author of the best-seller *The Book about Stretching* (translated into 18 foreign languages) and another Swedish original book about "Myths within sports, injuries and the locomotor system".

# Contents

# Part I

# Overview

# Introduction

The purpose of this book is to serve as a practical manual for doctors in the emergency room treating patients with injuries and disorders of the musculoskeletal system and as an orientation for nurses and other staff on modern management of these problems in an emergency or general practitioners' clinic.

The disposition is such that the chapter headings logically consist of the main complaint, for which the patient seeks emergency care (the symptoms). Under these headings the different diagnoses that could be appropriate in this connection are outlined, with the most important, and most common conditions marked with an *. The patients will – for obvious reasons – not come to the emergency clinic with a sign on their chest pointing out what diagnosis they are suffering from, for example, "meniscal rupture" and "hip dislocation".

Every actual disorder is then presented from only two aspects: (a) how to make the *diagnosis* and (b) what *treatment* should be given or is recommended in the emergency room. The illustrations are orientated towards practical management and realistic questions in the acute situation regarding treatment measures and examination findings of a kind which has to a great extent often been missing in the ordinary literature so far.

## Classification

To increase clarity, the reasons the patients came to the clinic can often be divided into three main categories: trauma, overload and overuse.
1. *Trauma* involves a direct and indirect impact cause of the injury.
2. *Overload* means that the strength of the actual tissue has been exceeded on one or a few occasions, e.g. rupture of the Achilles tendon.
3. *Overuse* is when an action has been performed by normal or low weight bearing but with many repetitions, and often in a monotonous pattern, e.g. in the case of a stress fracture.

S.-A. Sölveborn, *Emergency Orthopedics*,
DOI 10.1007/978-3-642-41854-9_1, © Springer-Verlag Berlin Heidelberg 2014

It is wise to make this distinction between overload and overuse since the treatment options for the subsequent disorders are often widely different.

## Fundamental Values

Basic behaviour and management in an emergency unit consists of the following fundamental principles:

1. *"The customer is always right"* – always behave politely and respectfully, listen carefully to the patient's thoughts and wishes.
2. Always take a thorough *patient history* – much of the solution to the problem is there, e.g. it has been shown that with the proper anamnestic information, 80 % of the diagnoses for knee and shoulder disorders can be made rather safely (even on the telephone!). Ask "When? Where? and How?" the complaint appeared and if the patient has had the same problem or a similar one previously.
3. *Examine the patient carefully* manually – Practice examination techniques continually. The patient history and examination status interpreted with good portions of knowledge and common sense are often better than sophisticated and expensive investigation techniques, e.g. magnet camera imaging (MRT), which are without doubt used more often than is absolutely necessary.
4. Try do develop the patient consultation in a way that the patient becomes *wiser* (and perhaps more knowledgeable than before about her/his situation) when she/he leaves the examination room. Always give *home instructions*, e.g. regarding physical activity, weight bearing and training instructions, so that the patient can take an active part in self-treatment to stimulate the healing process.
5. *Consult* the back-up on-duty doctor, colleague/specialist, instead of remaining doubtful about something – "there are no stupid questions, only stupid answers".
6. *Kindness and politeness* are often the keys to a good consultation; a smile could often be right, even in a difficult situation.
7. In the medical sphere and especially in a stressful environment like an emergency unit, it is important to remember that the doctor can sometimes *cure*, in most cases *relieve*, and always *comfort*!
8. *X-ray examinations are only shadows of reality* – a normal X-ray taken in casualty can give a false sense of security; analyse the X-ray findings carefully together with the clinical picture and consider taking an X-ray somewhat later, in the elective phase, or consider alternative examinations such as MRT, CT, scintimetry, etc. If the patient insists on having an X-ray taken, there is often no reason to refuse; sometimes, the X-ray can then also be performed after at a later point in time (see item 1 above about the customer).

# Major Orthopaedic Trauma

*In the primary assessment, an analysis of the trauma and a quick evaluation of the patient condition are included, advisably by the ATLS concept (Advanced Trauma Life Support) through the combination A-B-C-D-E. To secure vital life supporting functions, the A-B-C is the main priority, i.e. Airway (always secure a free airway first, this is the most urgent, and cervical spine control), Breathing (control of spontaneous breathing ability) and Circulation (control of pulse, heart activity and signs of circulatory shock with deteriorated cardiovascular function and consequent oxygen deficit). D and E represent a primary survey regarding Disability (reaction on speech/stimulation/pain) and Exposure (whole body examination) as well as Environment, respectively, in the following chronological order: Chest, Abdomen, Pelvis, Head (including neurology) and Skeleton. The vital functions are thus secured (with attention paid to the cervical spine) and neurological screening completed; after that the chest has the highest priority, followed by the head. People exposed to a major trauma have, on average, two to three body parts/ organ systems injured.*

## Injuries of the Pelvis

*Diagnosis.* Palpation and compression with respect to tenderness, hematoma (per rectum!), dislocations, sliding, also in vertical direction (since the most dangerous fractures have vertical instability/laxity) and from behind against the sacroiliaca joint. The fracture is stable if the pelvis ring is broken entirely or partly in only one place, but unstable if broken at least at two sites that leads to a sliding displacement/ translation between the two pelvis halves. Nerve injuries are not uncommon with unstable pelvis fractures.

*Treatment.* For unstable pelvis fracture, shock treatment is started; arrange as stable a fixation as possible with, e.g. girdle, coil banding or a vacuum mattress, and observe for possible injury to the large vessels (general circulatory

S.-A. Sölveborn, *Emergency Orthopedics*,
DOI 10.1007/978-3-642-41854-9_2, © Springer-Verlag Berlin Heidelberg 2014

compromise, large hematomas that can be of 2–3 litres size). Decision about urgent surgery with external fixation of the pelvis with anterior frame. Radiological mapping regarding skeleton and possible bleeding source (angiography). Also angiographic treatment with coiling could be indicated in selected cases.

## Spine Injuries

*Diagnosis.* Most often indirect trauma with distorsion and possibly rotation with compression of vertebral bodies that, with heavier violence, can disrupt and be pushed into the spinal canal. Fractures of vertebral arches incur a risk of instability and distraction injury to the spine marrow. Complete or incomplete transsectional lesions occur in spinal cord injuries, i.e. nerve function loss below the level of injury, above C4 paralysis of the breathing, at the C4-Th1 level tetraplegia and below this level paraplegia.

Injuries where the spinal cord is involved are, luckily enough, a relatively small portion of the spinal injuries.

The cervical spine and the thoracolumbar transitional zone are more often affected by injuries than the other parts. Observe the risk of cervical spine injuries after severe trauma to the head – often there are injuries to both head and neck! Injuries in the cervical spine and upper thorax can lead to loss of breathing function. Injuries to the cervical spine are common for severely injured patients; take caution when lifting, moving and examining. Avoid forward bending of the cervical spine! Observe and palpate the spine for dislocations, malformations, hematomas and tenderness at the spinous processes. Careful motion can provoke pain and crepitations. Check the ability to move the arms and the legs and the sensibility.

*Treatment.* Stabilise with stiff cervical collar and support, before and after the use of this, with, e.g. a towel roll in the cervical lordosis and cushions on both sides, alternatively use vacuum mattress. ATLS recommends manual stabilisation when removing the neck collar in case of intubation and clinical examination. Secure free airway, especially for patients with depressed consciousness. With signs of neurological deficits, high-dose corticosteroids can be given, but according to a different school of thought, steroids should not be administered. For unstable or dislocated injuries in the cervical spine, halo traction should be used (this can be done in local anaesthesia) with 12 kg of traction initially.

Shock treatment in circulatory compromise with primarily fluids and secondarily inotrops and vasopressors. Translation of a vertebra >3 mm and wedge angulation >11° indicates an unstable fracture, just as a combined anterior and posterior column injury does. Facet joint (sub)dislocation also suggests instability, even if the fracture cannot be visualised (ligamentous injury). Undisplaced stable fractures can be treated with a soft collar for 2–4 weeks, and if there is any doubt about the stability, the patient should be called back after 10 days for renewed X-ray with flexion-extension images. Open (penetrating) injuries should promptly receive antibiotics and be operated on, preferably at a neurosurgical unit.

## Extremity Injuries

*Diagnosis.* Systematic inspection of the extremities regarding presence of major bleeding, wounds or soft tissue injury and visible dislocation. Palpation on joints and diaphyses, cautious examination of movement to reveal pain reaction, tenderness, swelling and crepitations. Evaluate distal status with registration of vascular and nerve function distally from the injury (circulation, sensibility and motility). Observe signs of acute compartment syndrome like progressing pain, more firm muscle tissue in consistency (can become stiff like a board), weakness or inability to use the affected muscles and pain on passive stretch.

*Treatment.* Irrigate contaminated injuries with isotone saline fluid, stop bleeding with compression bandage. Cover injuries with sterile cloths. When needed, make preliminary gross morphological reduction to eliminate major fracture dislocations and joint dislocations, which, close to the time of injury (within 10–30 min), can be done even without anaesthesia or muscle relaxants. Always reduce by simultaneous traction in longitudinal axial direction, preferably together with a co-worker, who maintains resistance on the other side of the injury. Use slow and careful movements. First, neutralise gross angular dislocation and then gross rotational malposition. Keep the traction until the fixation/immobilisation is established. Give antibiotics early in case of open injuries with contamination or devitalized tissue. After traumatic amputation, there is as a rule astonishingly small or no bleeding (spasm of the arteries and fall of blood pressure), but risk of new arterial bleeding by shock treatment or movement of the patient. Disrupted and amputated body parts should be transported as sterile as possible, e.g. wrapped by compress in a sterile glove and/or in isotone saline solution in cold pack/ice bag. High priority for surgery when fractures with vascular or nerve injuries in spite of gross reduction, as well as open fractures. If circular plaster of cast is established primarily, it should always be cut up. Cast bandages should principally involve the joints on both sides of the fracture.

# Acute Soft Tissue Injuries

## (Strains and Contusions, e.g. in Sports)

## Measures

1. *Interrupt* the activity, e.g. sports exercise.
2. *High compression bandage* is immediately put directly on the skin with a fully outstretched elastic roller (corresponding to a pressure of 80 mmHg), possibly together with a pelot/adjusted disc on or around the injured area, kept on place for 15–20 min.
3. *Elevation*, where the heart is the reference level, preferably at least 50–60 cm above.
4. Change to *compression bandage* with moderate pressure after 15–20 min, i.e. with a halfway outstretched elastic roller (tip: stretch out the bandage fully, then reduce the traction to half the distance and wrap around, which corresponds to 40 mmHg), keep in place as long as swelling and/or pain still is experienced (usually 1–4 days). In this phase, cold treatment with ice bag or cold pack can be appropriate for pain relief and a certain amount of bleeding reduction through vascular contraction.
5. *Balanced/unloaded activity* early; motion without weight bearing can almost always be started immediately.

*Taping* of fingers and ankles may be performed for reasons of stabilisation, pain relief, stimulation of the proprioception and prevention of new distorsion, but never tape a swollen joint.

S.-A. Sölveborn, *Emergency Orthopedics*,
DOI 10.1007/978-3-642-41854-9_3, © Springer-Verlag Berlin Heidelberg 2014

# Part II

# Foot

# Foot Injuries

*Immediate measures: Elastic bandage (consider skin cleaning), elevation and X-ray*

## Contusion (including Subungual Hematoma) * S90.3/0

*Diagnosis.* Nearly always an impact or bump to the toes or from falling object. A hematoma under the big toenail can produce intense pain depending on the pressure.

*Treatment.* Evacuation with a straightened, tip-glowing paperclip directly through the nail, which often makes the blood squirt up and promptly relieves the pain.

## Toe Fracture (including Sesamoid Bone Fracture) * S92.4/5

*Diagnosis.* Most often direct trauma, with fracture more apparent hematoma discolouring (ecchymosis) than with contusion, but distal phalanx fractures often have simultaneous subungual hematomas. When a fracture of dig. 2–5 is suspected in an ordinary trauma situation, X-ray can in fact be refrained from. A safe sign is axial compression tenderness, with pressure in longitudinal direction.

*Treatment.* A displaced fracture of the proximal phalanx of the big toe should be reduced through traction and often fixed by pinning transcutaneously (or with open surgery). Undisplaced big toe fracture can be treated by so-called spica taping (overlapping taping along the entire big toe) for 2–3 weeks or just an elastic bandage together with wooden shoes or any other kind of broad and stable footwear.

S.-A. Sölveborn, *Emergency Orthopedics*,
DOI 10.1007/978-3-642-41854-9_4, © Springer-Verlag Berlin Heidelberg 2014

Fracture of the four lateral toes can, when necessary, be reduced by traction, taped or bound to the adjacent toe, and the patient is supplied with a steady shoe with a stable sole.

*Sesamoid bone fractures* often need special projection on X-ray or a scinti-graphic examination. Can occur after jumping from a significant height or as a stress fracture from overuse. Treatment with unloading insoles (also foam rubber with a shaped hole for the tender area) or a plaster cast with a cut-out around the bony protuberance for unloading when walking.

## Toe Joint Dislocation S93.1

*Diagnosis.* Direct trauma, often occurs in the MTP-joint with the proximal phalanx directed upwards dorsally. Pain and swelling can conceal the place of dislocation.

*Treatment.* Immediate reduction, which is often simple with moderate traction, may be done after toe base block with local anaesthetics, but also without it. If traction is initially not successful, hyperextend the toe with pressure on the meta-tarsal bone underneath. Avoid weight bearing initially, tape to the adjacent toe, eventually immobilisation up to 3 weeks.

## Metatarsal Bone Fracture * S92.3

*Diagnosis.* Common fractures, often squeeze/jam injuries, but also distorsion trauma and overload/overuse. Pain on weight bearing, swelling and restricted range of motion and typical tenderness at axial compression in longitudinal direction of the actual metatarsal. X-ray reveals the localisation for several types of injuries.

*Treatment. Metatarsal 5-base fractures:* In the so-called zone, an (see Fig. 1) avulsion fracture of the insertion of the peroneus brevis tendon is most common, can occur after supination and plantar flexion trauma, i.e. distraction fracture. Treated only with elastic bandaging, wide footwear, possibly unloading with crutch sticks and elevation in the earliest phase. In zone b is the sheer transverse or oblique fracture in the metaphysis-diaphysis transition area called (real) Jones fracture, which has a 40–50 % risk of non-union and is treated with plaster-of-cast without weight bearing for 4 weeks, then weight bearing in an orthosis additionally 2–4 weeks, if undisplaced. Surgery with pin fixation or intramedullar AO-screw if displaced. The diaphyseal fractures are located in zone c, where the *stress fractures* are most common, also called *march fractures*, most often on the meta-tarsal bone (2,) 3 or 4, i.e. as a consequence of repetitive overuse. Sometimes not

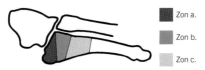

**Fig. 1** Fracture zones of the proximal part of the 5th metatarsal. *Zone a.* Avulsion of the tuberositas. *Zone b.* Jones' fracture. *Zone c.* Diaphyseal stress fracture

visible on plain X-ray if taken soon after the symptom debut (up to a week). In that case the X-ray has to be repeated after a week or an MRT or scintimetry is performed. March fractures are treated with stable shoes, preferably with an adequate high-posterior supporting wall and insoles. Adjusted weight bearing for 4 weeks is recommended.

*Diaphyseal metatarsal fractures* are otherwise often squeeze or crush injuries with significant soft tissue damage at the same time, in rare cases compartment syndrome. Treated with elastic bandage, elevation and reduction if more than 10° of angulation, sometimes open surgery including pin or screw fixation is needed to maintain the position, and this is valid for both fractures of the metatarsal shaft and the *subcapitular* ones of the collum. The latter type of MT 1 fracture or multiple metatarsal fractures are often unstable, have to be reduced and need pin stabilisation. A small plate fixation can be required for an unstable MT 1 fracture. Customary 1 week checkup with X-ray.

## Cuboid and Cuneiform Fracture S92.2

*Diagnosis.* Most often in combination with other injuries like dislocation in the TMT joint, isolated fractures are uncommon. Difficult to assess radiologically, CT is often needed.

*Treatment.* Elastic bandage, non-weight bearing for 3 weeks, cautious unloaded range of motion exercise early, then progressively increasing weight bearing.

## Dislocation of the Lisfranc Joint (Tarsometatarsal Joint, TMT) S93.3

*Diagnosis.* The TMT joint between the metatarsal bones and the cuboid and cuneiforms (see Fig. 2) is called the Lisfranc joint (complex) after the army surgeon of Napoleon, Jacques Lisfranc, who saw many dislocation injuries in this joint when horsemen fell off, were stuck in the stirrup and dragged after the horse! Nowadays they are mainly seen in high-energy trauma like traffic accidents, falls

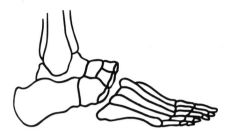

from great heights and industrial accidents, often in combination with other injuries
as fracture in the metatarsal bones (e.g. the base of MT 2), the cuboid or the
cuneiforms. The four lateral metatarsal bones are often dislocated laterally.

Heavy swelling, palpation, tenderness and pain on passive pronation and abduction
are typical findings. Computer tomography (CT) should be performed in a TMT
joint injury.

*Treatment.* Reduction necessary, this often has to be performed in open surgery,
since closed reductions are hard to perform. Fixation with pins and (cannulated)
screws is advised as casting alone after the reduction is advised against in view of
the difficulty in maintaining the position. Postoperatively, below-knee plaster-of-
cast for 10–12 weeks made removable to allow start of range of motion training
after 2 weeks. Gradually increase weight bearing during the plaster cast time, full
weight bearing after 10 weeks at the earliest, followed by individually made insoles.

## Navicular Fracture S92.2

*Diagnosis.* The most common type is an avulsion fracture (the attachment of
m. tibialis posterior), caused by flexion-eversion trauma to the middle foot, can
occur at the same time as a compression fracture of the cuboid ("nutcracker
fracture"). Longitudinal stress fractures and oblique fractures in dorsolateral to
plantar-medial direction occur, while a complete transverse fracture through the
entire navicular is uncommon.

High-energy trauma is often the cause, usually with other concomitant foot injuries.
Swelling dorsomedially, but the pain is often most marked in the plantar area.
Difficult to diagnose on X-ray, special rotated projections and/or CT often needed.

*Treatment.* Slightly displaced fractures and avulsions are treated with a plaster-of-
cast for 6 weeks allowing partial weight bearing initially, but transitional,
dislocated fractures should be reduced openly and fixed with compression

screw(s) through a dorsal incision. Postoperatively a below-knee plaster for about 10 weeks.

---

## Talus Fracture S92.1

*Diagnosis.* Caused by high-energy trauma such as traffic accidents (with axial load or fall from a significant height. Simultaneous dorsal extension of the foot produces a fracture through the *collum tali*, which in fact also can occur with ankle distorsion and is the most likely an associated injury to be neglected, since it is undisplaced. A great amount of swelling is common and inability of bearing weight because of the pain. The collum or the anterior parts of the *corpus tali* are most frequently affected. The greater dislocation/malposition, the greater risk of avascular necrosis (AVN) in the corpus that has a delicate blood supply (as has the caput femoris and os scaphoideum).

*Treatment.* Immediate fixation of the fracture with compression screws is alleged to decrease the risk of AVN. Doubtful if even undisplaced, collum tali fractures should be treated with a cast alone. Will need at least 8 weeks with a cast, even after surgery. The reduction manoeuvre for a dislocated collum tali fracture is by plantar flexion to exact position. If this is not achieved, open surgery with a stable fixation is indicated to allow early motion activity and partial weight bearing.
*Osteochondral fractures* of the corpus tali are relatively common and occur with distorsion trauma, can result in avascular necrosis and free body as a consequence and be a possible background to *osteochondrosis dissecans* (*OCD*). The treatment varies from unloading and/or plaster-of-cast to drilling and fixation of large detached fragments. *Processus lateralis tali fracture* can be missed since it is difficult to diagnose on plain X-ray, most often needs CT. If a larger fragment has been detached, reposition and fixation with pin or screw can be performed, or the fragment may need to be extracted.

---

## Dislocation in the Chopart Joint S93.3

*Diagnosis.* This joint complex includes the calcaneocuboid and the talonavicular joints. Like the talus dislocation, this is a rare injury. The mechanisms for these and for *subtalar dislocations* in general are forces in inversion with developing inward rotation and a pes equinus load (see Fig. 3). Concomitant rupture of the ligaments around the talus and the skin is common. The injury can be associated with a collum tali fracture, usually an open one. The foot can dislocate both in lateral and medial

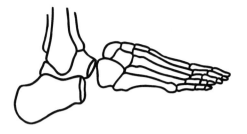

**Fig. 3** Dislocation of the Chopart joint

direction and the skin is always tilting markedly on the opposite side; heavy swelling is always present.

*Treatment.* Manual reduction in anaesthesia without delay by slow and firm traction in line with the deformity. Postreductional short below-knee plaster splint, swelling reduction and then early active motion exercises.

## Calcaneus Fracture * S92.0

*Diagnosis.* Most of these are caused by high-energy trauma like falls from a significant height in workplace accidents, from ladders and in traffic accidents. Young and middle-aged men are most commonly involved and relatively often bilaterally and a consequence of an axial load (be observant on simultaneous vertebral fracture!). Low-energy injury can be a cause, mainly in elderly patients with osteoporosis. Heavy swelling with a widening of the heel occurs fast and the bleeding is most evident on the plantar side; in 10 % of cases, a compartment syndrome in the foot develops. Severe pain at once that makes weight bearing impossible. Usually the fracture divides the calcaneus into an anterior medial part with the sustentaculum and a larger part including the tuber. About 75 % of the fractures are intra-articular. The degree of compression is measured by the so-called Böhler angle between the tuber calcanei and the talocalcaneal joints (see Fig. 4).

*Treatment.* Is influenced by the fracture appearance, bone quality, soft tissue injury, the activity level of the patient and the surgical experience of the treating orthopaedic surgeon. Immediate acute compression bandage, elevation and eventually cold treatment. Patients with undisplaced fractures are supplied with elastic bandage, non-weight bearing for 8–10 weeks, early unloaded motion exercises and individually made insoles. The somewhat elderly patient is treated with a below-knee cast. A well-cooperating patient may be supplied with a removable orthosis or just bandaging. There is no clear consensus regarding the indication for surgery, which is strengthened the more complex an intra-articular fracture is. On the other side, a too comminute fracture can be a contraindication for surgery. The soft tissue condition is critical for the decision if or when an operation should

**Fig. 4** The Böhler angle with
the anterior and posterior
facets of the calcaneus and the
superior edge of the
tuberositas as reference points

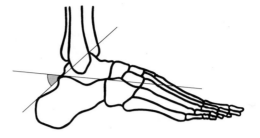

be performed; the swelling must be in regress; consequently surgery is often delayed 7–10 days. Incongruity in the joint surface correlates with an early development of arthrosis/osteoarthritis. Most patients need a life-long use of individually made shoe insoles.

# Foot Pain

## Arthritis (MTP and Toe Joints) *

*Diagnosis.* Can include reactive arthritis M02.9H, RA M06.9H, psoriatic arthritis M07.3H and crystal-induced arthritis M11.9H that in the proper sense of the diagnosis is a common name for different arthritis disorders, e.g. gout M10.0H and pyrophosphate arthritis M11.8H. The joints are warm, swollen and tender, and there is pain with movement. Take laboratory tests and X-ray. Reactive arthritis is often an oligoarthritis, affects adolescents and sometimes has eye and skin engagement. Take a history regarding recent GI or urogenital infections. With gout the MTP joint of the big toe often is intensely inflamed.

*Treatment.* Puncture and aspiration, joint fluid analysis and culture. Treat the underlying disease and, especially regarding the reuma-forefoot, prescribe orthopaedic supports like shoe insoles and orthotic devices. Wide shoes or sandals in the active phase (of disease). Possibly referral to a foot clinic. For gout, anti-inflammatory medication is prescribed initially and also colchicine can, at times, be indicated. By recurrences, prevention with allopurinol, but not the first time, unless the s-urate levels are distinctly elevated ("one time is no time"!).

## Hallux Rigidus M20.2

*Diagnosis.* Arthrosis/osteoarthritic development in the MTP joint 1 can be of both primary and secondary type, stiffness in the joint, especially and at an early stage in dorsal extension, that leads to difficulties in the foot lift-off phase during walking and a typical gait pattern with loading on the lateral side of the foot. Dorsal swelling due to osteophytes, often severe pain when weight bearing. Also painful gait without shoes. Sometimes hallux valgus occurs simultaneously.

S.-A. Sölveborn, *Emergency Orthopedics,*
DOI 10.1007/978-3-642-41854-9_5, © Springer-Verlag Berlin Heidelberg 2014

*Treatment.* Initially stretching in dorsal extension, then transverse bar shoe sole under the MTP joints, possibly local cortisone injection may be effective. Surgery could be an option, e.g. with debasing.

## Hallux Valgus M20.1

*Diagnosis.* There are several causes of the valgus angulation of the big toe, such as heredity, small and deforming shoes, foot hyperpronation and adductor contracture. Pain with pressure from the shoe at the medially protrubating metatarsal head 1 is the entirely dominating symptom with the formation of a pseudoexostosis, so-called bunion, that mainly consists of thickened and indurated soft tissue. Generally no pain when walking without shoes. The lateral deviation can be so great that the big toe rides over dig. 2. In that case there is also pain underneath the metatarsal head 2, as well as in the MTP joint 1. The grade can be measured (see Fig. 1) by the hallux valgus angle (HV) between the metatarsal 1 and the big toe or the intermetatarsal angle (IM) between the metatarsals 1 and 2. X-ray with exposure during weight bearing.

*Treatment.* Complete insoles with anterior pelot/disc and redression splint for use during night-time. Shoe selection with broad forefoot. Surgery with different osteotomy techniques (around 100 methods described!) when there is a wide valgus angle and/or severe subjective distress.

## Stress Fracture (Metatarsal and Navicular Insufficiency Fractures) * M84.3H

*Diagnosis.* Increasing pain on weight bearing after activity, most often diffuse pain initially, which later localises more distinctly. Occurs in many bones exposed to loading, but primarily in the diaphysis of the metatarsals 2, 3 or 5 (*march fracture*). Navicular stress fractures cause diffuse pain medially over the superior area of the foot and in the medial foot arch. Plain X-ray normal for 4–6 weeks if the fracture is localised diaphyseally (3–4 weeks if metaphyseal), but skeletal scintimetry shows positive finding considerably earlier as an MRI does (within 24 h!). A simple jumping manoeuvre, jump test, on the affected leg, will provoke a pinpoint localised pain reaction. Occurs in persons with predisposing factors like extrinsic types as incorrectly disposed training (most often a too rapid increase in dose or intensity), wrong shoes, smoking, etc. and/or by overuse or overload, especially in running or flexibility fitness sports. Local palpation tenderness, check with axial compression of the bone in question.

**Fig. 1** The hallux valgus
grade may be measured by the
hallux valgus angle (HV,
normally <15°) or
Intermetatarsal I–II angle
(IM, normally <9°)

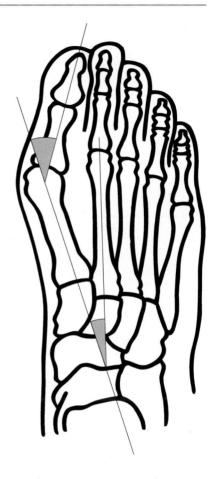

*Treatment.* For metatarsal bones a short time without weight bearing: however, the navicular needs more time. If detected early, changed, reduced or adjusted activity, all without immobilising. Preferably individual insoles that distribute the body weight more evenly over the foot. For athletes alternative training and then gradual return to sports under controlled rehabilitation and then wet-vest running in water and bicycling can be included. There is a certain small risk of delayed healing and development of pseudarthrosis, and surgery could then be indicated.

## Freiberg's Infarction/Osteochondrosis MTP M92.6

*Diagnosis.* Deformity in the metatarsal head with avascular necrosis subchondrally followed by a repair process including abundant osteophyte formation. Most often growing girls are affected usually dig. 2, so-called Köhler II.

*Treatment.* Adjustment of activity, avoiding impact to the foot and high-heeled shoes. Individual insoles and, for a couple of months, metatarsal transverse bar ("roll sole"). Surgical measures seldom indicated.

## Metatarsalgia M77.4

*Diagnosis.* Besides the above mentioned rare Freiberg's infarction and Mb Morton, metatarsalgia is a common name for widespread pain conditions on loading the metatarsal heads. Through downwards plantar protrusion, painful skin indurations, so-called *clavus,* are formed. Most patients try to avoid the pain by changing their gait pattern so that the load is transferred to the medial or lateral side of the foot.

*Treatment.* Individual shoe insoles and unloading discs/pads, always with an excavation for the painful area, but extirpation/resection of the clavus can also be necessary (make a cone-shaped excision); on some rare occasions, when there is prominence of the joint heads into the sole of the foot, more radical surgery may be necessary.

## Morton's Metatarsal Neuralgia * G57.6

*Diagnosis.* Most often not a real neuroma but rather a perineural fibrosis around the common digital nerve as it passes the metatarsal heads, due to repetitive irritation, usually affect the interstitium dig. 3–4, but the second and the other interspaces can also be involved (see Fig. 2). Mostly women in the age of 40–60 years (5:1 ratio compared to men). Usually starts with plantar pain, followed by radiating (burning) pain, dysesthesia and sometimes numbness in the affected toes. Pain is worse when shoes are worn, relieved by barefoot walking. Is a clinical diagnosis with palpation tenderness distally and between the metatarsal heads, where the patient often also experiences a radiating pain, sometimes in both distal and proximal direction. Can be provoked by vigorous dorsal extension of the toes.

**Fig. 2** Pain due to an
interdigital Morton's
"neuroma" (generally dig.
3–4 is affected, as seen here)
may be treated with an
injection between the
metatarsal heads

a

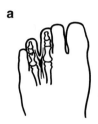

b

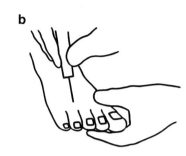

When the forefoot is squeezed from side to side, pain is provoked, and from time to time a recognisable click is experienced ("Mulder's click"). Only occasional sensory deficit. Management includes a standard X-ray.

*Treatment.* Individual shoe insoles/foot orthotics with anterior pads that lift and spread the metatarsal heads, shoes with broad anterior parts. Local cortisone injection (most often from the upper side, see Fig. 2) into the interstitium may be successful. In troublesome cases, surgery with neurotomy can be performed.

## Metatarsale-5 Enthesopathy M76.7

*Diagnosis.* Acute traumatic or insidious start of pain in the proximal part of the fifth metatarsal, made worse by walking, especially on hard surfaces and on stress of the fibularis muscles. Local tenderness over the proximal MT-5 end. Can be a tendon insertion pain (enthesopathy), an apophysitis or an avulsion fracture due to overuse of the fibularis (peroneus) muscles.

*Treatment.* Activity adjustment, some unloading, well-fitted shoes as support. Rehabilitation training (the fibularis muscles) if continued pain.

## Turf Toe M65.9H, M19.1H

*Diagnosis.* Redness and swelling of the great toe, often with a subungual haematoma, pain on all movements of the great toe, especially in dorsal extension. Occurs when the big toe is pressed forward in the shoe, e.g. at sudden deceleration friction on artificial turf and dorsal loading on the MTP-1. Tenderness at the dorsal side of the joint base of the great toe, and in time exophytes here gradually reduce range of motion, especially painful in dorsal extension. X-ray can show arthrosis/osteoarthritis including hallux rigidus and osteophytes dorsally.

*Treatment.* Shoe with fairly stiff sole for some time and space in front of the shoe with soft padding there. Taping to avoid vigorous dorsal extension should be tried. In later phases treatment as for hallux rigidus.

## Unguis Incarnatus L60.0

*Diagnosis.* Hangnail, ingrown toenail, where the nail grows downward–inward along the sides into the nail fold, most often caused by pressure from the outside due to tight shoes, but also a hereditary predisposition and a congenital incurved nail. In the first phase redness, swelling and tenderness along the lateral cuticle, then in phase 2 formation of an abscess with purulent or serous secretion, increased redness and tenderness and finally in phase 3 granulation tissue covers the nail, thereby inhibiting drainage. Can lead to recurrent infections, including *paronychia*.

*Treatment.* Initially shoe adjustment, open shoes or no shoes at all, trimming of the nail without cutting it to short. A compress can be inserted under the edge of the nail when the tenderness has diminished. On sign of infection, local antibiotic ointment or possibly peroral antibiotic medication.
If marked infection with abscess formation or recurrence, nail surgery is indicated with avulsion of the entire or preferably a part of the nail, as in König's operation, where about ¼ of the nail is removed through a longitudinal cut through the skin, made in toe-base block anaesthesia.

## Tarsal Tunnel Syndrome G57.5

*Diagnosis.* The most common nerve entrapment in the hindfoot, where n. tibialis posterior is compressed just below the lower edge of the medial malleolus in the tarsal tunnel, almost always with a calcaneovalgus-pronated foot. Often diffuse and intermittent symptoms with pain over the medial part of the ankle radiating to the foot arch, but can also go upwards towards the calf. Numbness and paraesthesia that are exasperated by walking or dorsal extension of the foot. Tinel's sign is positive when tapping on the nerve course or compression of the nerve for 30 s. Pain and cramps in the foot arch can occur, as well as night-time dysesthesias. Two-point discrimination can be decreased in the foot. The diagnosis is clinical; EMG can support it, but is not necessary.

*Treatment.* Foot orthotics to compensate for hyperpronation. Local cortisone injection is usually not successful. In persistent cases, surgery with neurolysis and tarsal tunnel release may be indicated.

## Plantar Fascialgia (Including "Heel Spur") * M72.2

*Diagnosis.* Very common painful condition, occurs from the tendinous insertion of the plantar fascia into the calcaneus, as a matter of fact incorrectly named "heel spur". A finding on X-ray of an exostosis/spur on the spot is of no importance, since this is commonly present also among entirely symptom-free persons. A preferable and better describing name is plantar fascia insertalgia. May start spontaneously, but most likely after overuse, caused by running (in fact the most common cause of heel pain in athletes) or walking longer distances, and hyperpronation of the hindfoot can be the reason behind it. Typical pain pattern with initial pain on weight bearing after getting up in the morning, or after rest, often decreasing within a matter of minutes and then returning during the day on continued walking/running. There is a tendency of chronicitation with pain possibly persevering for one or several years. The most tender spot is classically at the medial plantar and anterior part of the calcaneus when palpating from the foot arch, but also palpation under the more central part of the heel and further anteriorly along the plantar fascia can provoke pain. The diagnosis is clinical and not from X-ray, but this can rule out other causes.

*Treatment.* Practically always nonsurgical with activity adjustment and full-size insoles with excavation for the painful area. A special "cup" that keeps the heel pad together and at the same time has an excavation for the medio-anterior part of the heel may also be motivated. Studies have shown good effect of stretching techniques both for the plantar fascia as such (dorsal extension stretch in the MTP joints), but also for the Achilles tendon (dorsal extension for the entire ankle, see Fig. 3). Stiffness in the Achilles tendon increases the tension of the plantar fascia during walking. Night splint for static stretching of the plantar fascia during 1–2 months has also shown good results. Local cortisone injection at punctum maximum near the bone can often have a strikingly good (although at times only temporary, 1–2 months) effect. Taping often gives good pain reduction with a technique that also unloads the fascia on weight bearing. Shock wave therapy (ECSWT) has in some studies shown nice results. Surgery with release of the fibrotic insertion area for very resistant cases has also been described with good results, but is more controversial.

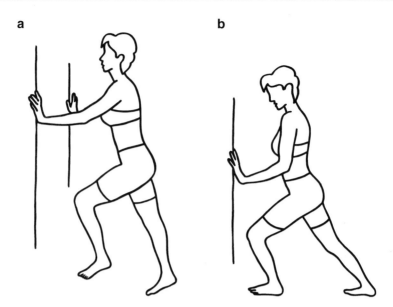

**Fig. 3** Stretching for the right Achilles tendon with dorsal extension of the ankle joint. *Phase a*: Muscle contraction by toe standing/heel raise for 6–10 s. *Phase b*: Stretching in end position kept still for 15–20 s with hand support rather low to get better relaxation

## Haglund–Severs Disease M92.8

*Diagnosis. Calcaneus apophysitis*, with pain posteriorly in the heel at the insertion of the Achilles tendon after overload in prepubertal children, most often boys, especially in connection with sports and play with overuse risk through repetitive microtrauma from traction at the apophysis via the Achilles tendon. Evidently associated with moderate idiopathic pes cavus–varus. The pain can increase with time and cause a slight limp. Palpation tenderness on compression towards the insertion of the Achilles tendon. X-ray shows irregularity in the epiphysis line, but is not diagnostic.

*Treatment.* Activity adjustment and the use of impact-reducing insoles, sometimes outlasting of the posterior heel grip of the shoe. Heel heightening of the shoe a short time for pain relief and then commencement of careful stretching of the Achilles tendon. Never an indication for cortisone injection. Good prognosis, no long-term problems.

## Os Trigonum Impingement M89.2

*Diagnosis.* Separate ossification centre behind the talus as an extra bone that could be subjected to impingement like a hazelnut in a pair of nutcrackers between the calcaneus and the posterior part of tibia on forced plantar flexion of the foot. Pain on both active and passive plantar flexion, like the "en pointe" position in ballet. Can affect vessels n. tibialis posterior and flexor hallucis longus. In junction with the talus that gets an elongation posteriorly, this phenomenon is called *Stieda* protuberance. Both the os trigonum and the Stieda protuberance can be fractured.

*Treatment.* An injection with corticosteroid may possibly be tried, but if the complaint is significant, a surgical extirpation of the bone part has to be performed.

## Achilles Insertalgia (including Achilles Bursitis) * M77.5, M71.5

*Diagnosis.* Can be a pain condition at the insertion of the Achilles tendon at the calcaneus and/or in the deep retrocalcaneal bursa in the Kager triangle (which can result in a bulging on both sides of the Achilles tendon) or the superficial bursa between the skin and the heel bone ("pump bump"). It usually affects middle-aged and elderly persons, but is also a common overuse disorder in sports. The insertion can become calcified and thus visible on X-ray. Local swelling and tenderness, pain by active and passive dorsal extension of the foot.

*Treatment.* Change of shoes (e.g. to shoes without posterior heel grip), outlasting of the posterior heel grip and stretching of the Achilles tendon (see Fig. 3, page 28) are always included. Puncture with aspiration and a local cortisone injection in the bursa, but not to the tendon, can be tried. In the most acute phase, local anti-inflammatory ointment (gel) is indicated, applied by massage twice a day for 7–10 days. Full-size foot orthotics for avoidance of shear forces to the Achilles tendon.

## Heel Pad Syndrome M70.8

*Diagnosis.* A consequence of either an acute, forceful impact injury or repetitive traumata towards the heel such as running on hard surfaces or football played with insufficiently impact-reducing shoes. Damage to the fat pad ("tread through") and the sophisticated impact-absorbing structure with connective tissue septa and spiral fibres that runs between the subcutis and into the calcaneus. Pain on weight bearing, tenderness and often reduced fat substance over the heel bone is evident.

*Treatment.* Shock-absorbing insoles, possibly foot orthotics ("cup") with higher side brims that press the heel pad together. Activity adjustment, some unloading during the most acute phase.

# Foot Wounds

## Traumatic Wound S91.3

*Diagnosis.* Mostly simple causes like direct trauma, squeeze injuries (e.g. subungual hematoma), sharp or pointed objects, etc. Sometimes a *subungual exostosis*, especially at the distal phalanx of the big toe, can be a causal factor. Be aware that the foot region can be contaminated very often by bacteria.

*Treatment.* Careful cleaning, all wounds can be generously rinsed with ordinary tap water – lavish (in fact there are more infections related to saline fluid dressings!). Important to remove possible asphalt road rash. If a foreign body is suspected and difficult to identify, apply a local anaesthetic and, in a blood-free field, expose the wound clearly, e.g. by an elongated incision or a help incision in the skin. Skin defects up to 1½ cm in diameter can granulate if they are covered, e.g. with lenient Mepitel dressing (has a silicone surface). Bigger defects should be covered by a partial dermal transplantation. The own skin is the best bandage, even if it is detached (decollement injury). If tendons are exposed in the wound: cover and keep moist. Use hydrogel ("moist on gallipot"), hydrofibre (Aquacel) and plastic compress (Solvaline). Tetanus prophylaxis should be considered. Avoid sensitization to antibiotics by abstaining from all local treatment with antibiotic-containing wound products.

## Diabetic Ulcers * E10.5

*Diagnosis.* Foot complications such as ulcers, infection, deformity and ischemia affect hardly 10 % of the diabetics; the greatest problem is with type 2 diabetics over 60 years of age. The patient's whole situation must be evaluated from a multidisciplinary perspective. The neuropathy leads to that ordinary warning signal on overload, and trauma is not recognised so that ulcers, chaps or infections are not

S.-A. Sölveborn, *Emergency Orthopedics*,
DOI 10.1007/978-3-642-41854-9_6, © Springer-Verlag Berlin Heidelberg 2014

detected in the early phase. Of the patients with wounds, 70–100 % have neuropathy. Areas with lack of hair and colour changes are signs of ischemia, check the foot pulses, if possible measure toe blood pressure (limit 30 mmHg, ankle pressure 50 mmHg indication for angiography). Observe that no ulcers are free of bacteria! Culture (from the wound edge or deep centrally and blood culture if suppressed general state of health or fever), but the mere presence of bacteria is not an indication for antibiotic therapy (with the exception of streptococcus type A), in the same way that presence of ulcer as such is not either. By culture you get another spectrum than for nondiabetics, often gram-negative *Staphylococcus aureus* and even anaerobes. More than 50 % lack the classic signs of a severe infection with increase of CRP/SR and fever. Most patients just feel a dull discomfort with a slight pain; with superficial infections there is a lack of pain. Deep infections are most commonly plantar; dorsal abscesses on the foot can have a plantar origin. Liberal indication for X-ray with foot ulcers (osteitis, insufficiency fracture, osteopathia).

*Treatment.* More than 80 % of the infected diabetes ulcers need surgical intervention; deep infection incurs about a 50 % risk of amputation. It is as important with incision *and drainage* as with choice of antibiotics. General principle: Leave the ulcer open! Avoid local antibiotics. *Superficial* ulcers (not contamination) are primarily treated with flucloxacillin 750 mg 1–2 × 2 per os, if hypersensibilisation occurs or insufficient effect: clindamycin 150–300 mg × 3 per os. Do not continue if the infection is healed, evaluate continuously at 10–14 days at the latest. An acute *deep* infection is treated intravenously, and with surgery, in the first place with cephalosporins or ciprofloxacin 200–300 mg × 2 IV and metronidazole 400 mg × 3 per os. Change to per oral treatment if the clinical picture is mitigated and in accordance with culture results. Revision/resection of devitalised tissue and bone that impedes healing; almost always a wider resection, than first expected, is needed. If drained surgically, gentamicin pellets locally for 1–2 weeks is recommended. Wound dressing change several times daily with a well-pressed moist saline compress. Referral to a diabetes foot therapist. Do not choose occlusive treatment – risk of maceration and ulcer expansion. Immobilisation is of importance, often by plaster-of-cast with fenestration (be aware that the swelling does not bulge out and lead to edge injuries in the skin) to make bandaging possible, but remove the cast at once if there is any deterioration. The cast therapy is a good method for healing of an ulcer, but requires long time, often 6 months for a large ulcer on the sole of the foot. Orthotic device can be used as an alternative. Unloading insoles should be considered for weight distribution over the foot. Dry, black, ischemic toe necroses should not be treated, but left for spontaneous amputation (mummification). Consult a vascular surgeon before amputation is considered, supplementary treatment for vascular disease: acetylsalicylic acid (aspirin) in tablet form 75 mg × 1. General treatment efforts: aggressive treatment of oedema (compression bandaging, pump boot, possibly diuretics), instructions for physical activity (ergometer bicycle, unloaded motion exercises), shoe checkup so that they are not too tight (the majority of the diabetic ulcers are caused by unfit/

unsuitable shoes; they should be ½ cm wider than the feet), smoking cessation and antihypertensive therapy.

## Arteriosclerotic/Ischemic Ulcer * I70.2

*Diagnosis.* A differential diagnosis to diabetic foot ulcer. More intense pain reaction, deteriorates on elevation.

*Treatment.* Increased physical activity engaging feet and legs, vascular surgeon consultation. Ulcer bandaging after cleaning and wound revision, debride down to healthy, bleeding tissue and maintain moisture. Protect the ulcer and prevent from microbiological contamination; if not healed within 6 weeks, contact should be made with a local wound care clinic.

## Varicose Leg Ulcer I83.9
See section "Venous Insufficiency" (observe the treatment with compression) under the chapter "Swelling of the Foot and Ankle".

# Part III
# Ankle

# Swelling of the Foot and Ankle

## Venous Insufficiency * I87.2

*Diagnosis.* Most often visible varices and thrombophlebitis, vascular oedema, sometimes of the pitting oedema type, often brownish discolorations in the skin.

*Treatment.* Compression therapy of different modalities, always elastic bandaging and instructions for increased physical activity. Weight reduction when appropriate. Consideration of surgical measures regarding the varices.

## Deep Venous Thrombosis (DVT) I80.3

*Diagnosis.* In most age groups, but increased risk over 40, similar frequency between the genders. Grave prognosis if untreated. Among other risk factors extended immobilisation (e.g. with plaster-of-cast), previous DVT or pulmonary embolism, adiposity, congestive heart failure and infarction, fractures of the hip or leg, knee and hip arthroplasties, hip fracture surgery, multiple trauma, long journeys, contraceptive pills, pregnancy, infection, stroke and malignancy could be mentioned. Most begin in the veins of the calf with poor reflow. Most patients are asymptomatic; generally there are a few symptoms: pain and swelling on the upper foot, ankle and lower leg; phlebitis is also possible. Swelling that remains in spite of elevation. Tenderness, redness, certain induration and increased venous stasis picture. Pain in the calf with exasperation on dorsal extension of the foot (= Homan sign positive, but not fully conclusive for thrombosis). Venography (phlebography) is the golden standard method; also ultrasound Doppler is an adequate option. Thrombosis in, or proximal of, the popliteal fossa carries a 50 % risk of pulmonary embolisation.

S.-A. Sölveborn, *Emergency Orthopedics*,
DOI 10.1007/978-3-642-41854-9_7, © Springer-Verlag Berlin Heidelberg 2014

*Treatment.* Transfer to an internal medicine unit for immediate anticoagulation therapy.

## Heart Failure * I50.9

*Diagnosis.* Distal swelling of pitting oedema type, i.e. when pits remain in the skin after finger pressure, most commonly bilateral. Look for heart symptoms like band-shaped pain and pressure over the chest.

*Treatment.* Referral to an internal medicine unit.

## Ankle Injury (Distorsion/Sprain, Fracture) *

See chapter "Ankle Injuries".

# Ankle Injuries

*First measures for severe ankle injuries: Preliminary reduction at once when necessary, elastic bandage, elevation, consideration for the skin, examine distal status, transport splint and quickly to X-ray!*

## Ankle Distorsion * S93.4

*Diagnosis.* The most common diagnosis in emergency units receiving orthopaedic patients. Each day one in 10,000 inhabitants is injured; 2/3 of the ankle injuries at the emergency units are from sports. It is also the most common sports injury in general, 15–20 % of all injuries in football, handball, volleyball and orienteering, but often much higher incidence in basketball. Recurrences are common (in soccer football 67–75 %), indicating insufficient rehabilitation of previous injuries, often delayed healing process (50 %). Often residual symptoms on strenuous activity and weight bearing (40 %) more than 1 year after the trauma. Incidence peak at 15–25 years of age, right = left in the distribution. The ligament fibulotalare anterius (FTA) is injured in 87 %, "all" cases are in principal total ruptures, partial injuries are rare and combination injury is more common if there is a previous ankle injury, and these cause more swelling and tenderness. Of all ankle injuries, 85 % occur on inward rotation–supination + plantar flexion. Medial injuries more uncommon, ligamentum deltoideum is one of the strongest ligaments in the body (has three portions), and an oblique movement axis in the ankle joint makes the lateral side more prone to sprain injury. Examine as early as possible also to differentiate against fractures. Injuries to the *syndesmosis* and *physis* must not be overlooked. The syndesmosis consists of the anterior and posterior tibiofibular ligaments (TFA + TFP). Always perform an X-ray on children and the (biological) elderly, but all others need not to go to X-ray unless they are tender on palpation over the lateral or medial malleoli (the Ottawa rules have 100 % sensitivity). It is smart to palpate the medial malleolus first, then the fibula along the *posterior* line from the proximal to the distal end (since the FTA ligament attaches anteriorly).

S.-A. Sölveborn, *Emergency Orthopedics*,
DOI 10.1007/978-3-642-41854-9_8, © Springer-Verlag Berlin Heidelberg 2014

**Fig. 1** Laxity test of the
stability of the ankle joint,
so-called anterior drawer test:
With a distinct grip around
the heel, the foot is pulled
forward anteriorly (and
counteraction at the lower
leg). With a simultaneous
traction this is also the
reduction manoeuvre for
displaced ankle fractures

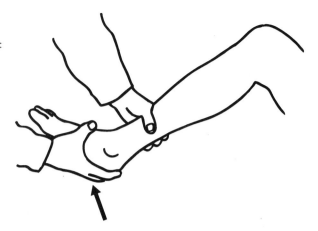

Syndesmosis tests: "Squeeze" sign, compression of the diaphyses from side to side in the lower leg to elicit distal pain (= indirect pain) and (forceful) outward rotation sign and laxity side to side (transition sideways). X-ray the entire fibula (to reveal a high fibula fracture) if a syndesmosis injury is suspected. Laxity test: "Anterior drawer" sign in 10° of plantar flexion (see Fig. 1), but this is often not conclusive in the most acute phase.

*Treatment.* (1) Full compression bandage (maximally drawn out elastic bandage) for 20 min. (2) Elevation (60 cm over the level of the heart). (3) Compression bandage (with half out-drawn elastic bandage), *eventually* in combination with ice/cold pack. (4) Early weight bearing, unloaded motion exercises straight away. (5) Possibly mobilisation with ankle orthosis (or ankle taping) after 24 h. (6) To physiotherapist within 2 days for rehabilitation exercises, taping or testing of orthosis. If high stability is demanded, e.g. in sports, supporting bandage with tape or orthosis for at least 3 months. Home programme of ankle rehabilitation with three components: (1) Strength exercises of the heel-raise type. (2) Flexibility training with dorsal extension stretching (*as* Achilles tendon stretching; see Fig. 3 of chapter "Foot Pain", page 28). (3) Coordination and balance training, daily for at least 6–8 weeks.

## Ankle Fracture: * Lateral S82.6, Medial S82.5, Bimalleolar or Trimalleolar S83.8

*If dislocated, perform a reduction (see* Fig. 1) *immediately before X-ray. Surgery if >2 mm of dislocation.*

*Diagnosis.* Classification according to AO (Danis–Weber, Müller) with respect to the lateral malleolus: *A-type* (below the joint space), after a supination trauma, generally no syndesmosis rupture, stable; *B-type* (at the joint space level) includes external rotation, has syndesmosis rupture in 50 %, thus often stable too; *C1-type* (proximal of the joint space) from pronation has 100 % syndesmosis rupture, as does the *C2-type*, where the medial malleolus is fractured, unstable. Observe the congruence of the ankle joint!

*Treatment.* Successful treatment is based on reduction to congruence in the ankle joint and the maintenance of it. Dislocated fractures are immediately reduced; *tip*: Flex the knee to reduce the traction in the calf muscles (see Fig. 1, page 40). C-type fractures (unstable) should be operated on without delay (within 6–8 h), but wait if the skin is tense until the swelling is reduced. Elastic bandage and elevation in the meantime. Moreover, surgery if the dislocation in the fracture is >2 mm. Otherwise, either a lower leg cast with the foot in plantigrade position (= 0° in the ankle joint!) or, if there is a fairly stable unimalleolar fracture, ankle orthosis of the Walker boot type for 4–6 weeks. X-ray check after 1 week. Gradually increasing weight bearing for stable fractures. Minimally or non-dislocated fractures, fissures, may be unloaded with crutch sticks for 3 weeks and be supplied with elastic bandage or ankle orthosis of stirrup type. Avulsion fracture at the tip of the lateral malleolus is equivalent to a ligament injury, a sprain. Consider if the ankle fracture could have been precipitated by osteoporosis (see the chapter "Osteoporosis"). Syndesmosis injury can occur even without a malleolar fracture.

Isolated fracture of the lateral malleolus at the syndesmosis level (SE 2-type according to the Lauge–Hansen classification) or below this level (SA 1-type) with 2 mm displacement at the most, thus can be treated with a lower leg cast boot or alternatively a stirrup bandage for 6 weeks.

## Ankle Fractures in Children * S82.6/S82.5/S82.8

*Diagnosis.* Indirect rotation trauma, most often in the distal tibia, but there can be an isolated fibular injury. The growth plate – the physis – involved in the Salter–Harris classification (see Fig. 2), where the type II fracture is the most common. Two additional special types occur: Tillaux fracture (in children ≥12 years of age) with a square fragment from the anterior lateral part of the distal tibia epiphysis (S-H type III) and triplane fracture with fracture lines in three planes.

*Treatment.* Acute reduction to exact position in general anaesthesia with the knee in flexion and grip around the heel and upper side of the foot (see Fig. 1, page 40). If this cannot be achieved for Salter–Harris type III and IV injuries, as well as for Tillaux and triplane fractures, surgery with open reduction and, generally, osteosynthesis.

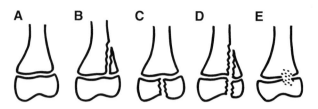

**Fig. 2** The Salter–Harris classification of physeo-related injuries (from *left*): (**A**) Physeolysis without fracture, (**B**) Physeolysis with a metaphyseal bone fragment (Holland's sign), (**C**) Intraarticular epiphyseal fracture and physeolysis, (**D**) Intraarticular epiphyseal fracture that intersect the physis and continues up in the metaphysic, and (**E**) Compression injury to the physis (rare, initially not visible on X-ray)

Salter–Harris type I and II injuries with <2 mm displacement: plaster-of-cast for 4–6 weeks depending on the age of the child (so also postoperatively). Physiolysis fracture through the lateral malleolus: lower leg cast for 3 weeks. X-ray post-operatively and postreductionally after 1 week and after half a year in view of the risk of growth disturbance.

## Pilon Fracture (Tibia Plafond Fracture) S82.3

*Diagnosis.* This distal lower leg fracture is a special type of ankle fracture (in the "ceiling") with compression and fragmentation, so that the fracture engages the joint surface of the tibia. Comminute fracture type after high-energy trauma such as motor vehicle accidents or falls from a significant height. Most often heavy swelling and for mapping will sometimes tomography be needed.

*Treatment.* Immediate rough reduction manoeuvre (see Fig. 1, page 40) after anaes-thesia, anti-swelling with strict elevated position, elastic bandage and stabilisation with a temporary cast splint. Attention paid to the risk of acute compartment syndrome. Surgery after removal of swelling, including reconstruction of the joint surface. No weight bearing for 2–3 months.

## Achilles Tendon Rupture * S86.0

See the chapter "Lower Leg Injuries".

## Fibular Tendon Dislocation (Peroneal Tendon Dislocation) M67.8

*Diagnosis.* Rare disorder, predominantly affects individuals between 10 and 25 years of age. Usually traumatic origin from an ankle distorsion classically caused by skiing, especially on contraction in plantar flexion and eversion, when the peroneal retinaculum is torn so that one or both fibular (peroneal) tendons dislocate from their tunnel below and behind the lateral malleolus. Often a lash is experienced, either with or without pain, and swelling can occur. In predisposed individuals with a shallow sulcus, where the tendons glide, the phenomena can occur spontaneously. In more than half of the patients, the disorder will be permanent with recurrent instability as a consequence, including a snapping discomfort when the tendon glides anteriorly up on the malleolus. The patient can often reproduce the (sub)dislocation with muscle contraction in dorsal ankle extension and foot eversion, and you can feel how the tendon clicks forward. In the acute phase the presentation is similar to an ordinary lateral ankle ligament injury, which it may be confused with X-ray. In 15–50 % of the cases, there is an avulsion fracture at the posterior edge of the malleolus, which is a pathognomonic sign of the diagnosis.

*Treatment.* Initially compression bandage and then ankle orthosis for 4 weeks. In later phases usually surgery has to be performed (successful in about 90 %) with, e.g. retinaculum reconstruction and deepening of the tendon sulcus. Special taping could be tried with a pelot/disc-like arrangement to keep the tendons in place behind the lateral malleolus.

# Ankle Pain

## Posttraumatic Synovial Impingement * M65.9H

*Diagnosis.* Synovial irritation that persists in varying frequency and intensity with tendency of swelling, so that, in the typical cases, impingement occurs with sudden pain attacks as a consequence ("like a knife into the joint"). Much more common condition than expected. On arthroscopy there are often synovial protrusions of lip-like or sea-grass appearance, sometimes also fibrous bands (plica formation) or meniscoid lesions. Palpation tenderness, especially against the ankle joint anteriorly. Synovitis reactions can be seen without trauma in collagenoses, reactive arthritis, gout, RA and similar conditions, as well as with instability.

*Treatment.* Elastic bandaging and alternative activity (e.g. swimming and bicycling). Ankle joint puncture (see Fig. 1) can be appropriate, anti-inflammatory medication, as well as possibly a cortisone injection into the joint, if you can be sure that the joint surfaces are intact (N.B. the collagen destructive effect of local corticosteroids). Ankle arthroscopy with synovial resection for the more persistent cases most often has good results. An ankle rehabilitation programme with strength, flexibility and balance exercises is important.

## Osteochondrosis (Dissecans) Tali * M93.2H

*Diagnosis.* Osteochondral lesions are in fact common after ankle distorsions, especially after high-energy trauma with an impact or translation injury, such as jumping or running at a considerable speed, but are often not detected until much later, e.g. when an X-ray is performed due to persistent pain problems (and when X-ray at the time for the original trauma in fact was normal). The upper part of the talus can be affected by compression injuries, most often the medial area quite central on the so-called talar dome. There can be a grading from mild compression

S.-A. Sölveborn, *Emergency Orthopedics*,
DOI 10.1007/978-3-642-41854-9_9, © Springer-Verlag Berlin Heidelberg 2014

**Fig. 1** Ankle joint puncture is performed in the anterior lateral (or medial) third; the arterial passage in the central part must be avoided (see also the chapter "Basic Injection Techniques")

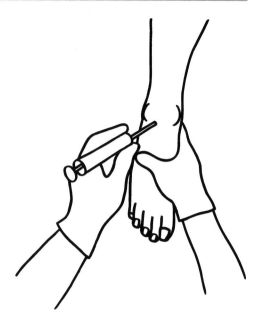

(also stress fracture like) of cartilage and subchondral bone to a more severe injury with a detached fragment, which can form a free body in the joint. The cartilage can survive due to diffusion, but an *avascular necrosis* or a *loose body* could consequently develop. On X-ray subchondral cyst formation can be seen, on MRI oedema in the talus and on isotope scintimetry: focally increased uptake. Such a traumatic osteochondral lesion is regarded as one of several causes behind *osteochondrosis dissecans* (formerly with the inappropriate name osteochondritis dissecans – as there is no inflammation present), which also can occur without a known trauma. Certain pain on weight-bearing and joint effusion can be present, as well as varying pain on flexion–extension movement, but translational pain is a constant finding. Stiffness and locking (mechanical by a loose body) can occur, but pain on palpation need not be present.

*Treatment.* For milder forms reduction of impact (bumps, sudden pressure loading) to enable healing of the lesion centre during 6–12 weeks. In the more advanced stages, extraction or fixation of the bone cartilage fragment (ossicle) in combination with drilling of the underlying tissue, so-called Pridie drilling, which can be done arthroscopically and gets 70–90 % of the patients back to normal ankle function.

Bone transplantation into the bone defect can be considered via arthrotomy (and osteotomy through the medial malleolus).

## Loose Body in the Joint M24.0H

*Diagnosis.* Intermittent mechanical and/or pain-related lockings in the typical cases. Can be combined with an osteochondral defect in the talus or osteophytes on the anterior border of the tibia (gradually also on the talus) in so-called footballer's ankle (with anterior impingement). Both bony and chondral fragments can occur.

*Treatment.* Arthroscopic extraction or refixation of the loose body.

## Osteochondral Defect M93.2H

See section "Osteochondrosis (Dissecans) Tali" above.

## Subdislocating Fibular (Peroneal) Tendon M67.8

See the chapter "Ankle Injuries".

## Posterior Tibial Tendon Rupture/Tendalgia S96.2/M76.8

*Diagnosis.* This tendon rupture is rare, but occurs in "older" athletes down towards the attachment/insertus, which is remarkably wide and includes the navicular bone, all the three cuneiforms and the metatarsals 2, 3 and 4. The rupture can occur by ankle distorsion and then most often behind the medial malleolus, but also closer to the attachment at the navicular bone. The most common cause of injury is jumping in connection with gym work-out in a middle-aged woman (40–60 years). In most cases there is such a traumatic episode, but there can also be a more insidious course with pain down to the attachment area – *tibialis posterior syndrome*. In the typical case increasing medial foot pain with progressive flatfoot deformity (when the tibialis posterior does not manage to keep the foot arch in position). Palpation tenderness along the tendon and a defect from total rupture, most common just distal to the medial malleolus, swelling. The patient cannot perform heel raising to tiptoe position, and a typical valgus position is seen in the hindfoot/heel, hyperpronation with "too many toes sign" (three or more toes could be seen lateral to the lateral malleolus when standing if looked at straight from behind). There may also be pain in the lateral part of the hindfoot due to impingement of the calcaneus against the fibular tip. The muscle function can be examined if the patient, with the foot in supination, tries to resist the examiners attempt to transfer the foot into pronation. Clinical diagnosis can be verified by MRI or ultrasound.

*Treatment.* Initial unloading, customised (individual) foot insoles with medial support and hindfoot-stabilising orthosis. Local cortisone injection should never be given. For total rupture, surgery with suture and possibly augmentation of the tendon (or tendon reconstruction) is usually necessary, thereby also aiming to prevent the development of a very troublesome flatfoot.

## Ankle Osteoarthrosis ("Osteoarthritis") M19.0H/M19.1H

*Diagnosis.* Most common in elderly with a previous ankle fracture or hereditary predisposition. Can have sudden pain attacks due to synovial impingement, as well as swelling tendency and restriction of range of motion. X-ray, which for the ankle "always" should be taken with the patient in standing, weight-bearing position, verifies the diagnosis.

*Treatment.* Elastic bandage (counteracts swelling and stimulates the proprioception), alternative activity, short course(s) with anti-inflammatory medication, crutch sticks for partial support and ankle rehabilitation programme (strength, flexibility and balance exercises). In advanced cases arthrodesis or arthroplasty with an artificial joint prosthesis.

## Achilles Tendalgia, Achilles Paratendinosis * M76.6

See the chapter "Lower Leg Pain".

## Referred Pain from the Back (Nervus Fibularis/Peroneus Communis and Spf.) * M54.3

*Diagnosis.* Compression of a nerve root in the lumbar spine, most often L5–S1, can be the only or a persistent symptom, presents itself by numbness in the corresponding dermatome and weakness in the foot, e.g. as a consequence of a disc hernia, but the cause could also be an entrapment of the fibular/peroneal communis or superficialis nerves. Paresthesia, hyperesthesia and sensibility deterioration can be noted.

*Treatment.* Avoid local pressure in the area; this irritates the nerve even more. Treatment of the primary cause lumbosacrally, for a distal aetiology surgery with neurolysis can be indicated.

# Part IV

# Lower Leg

# Lower Leg Injuries

## Pilon Fracture S82.3

See the chapter "Ankle Injuries"

## Tibial and Fibular Fractures * S82.2/S82.3/S82.1

*Diagnosis.* Lower leg fractures caused by direct trauma are most often of transverse type, while those caused by indirect trauma are oblique or spiral fractures. High-energy injuries such as traffic accidents often result in comminute fractures as well as extensive injuries to the soft tissue. Be aware of the possibility of acute compartment syndrome! An isolated tibial fracture is more common in children and young people than in elderly, who most often have both the tibia and the fibula fractured. Problem with weight bearing, pain with movement, swelling, palpation tenderness and sometimes visible dislocation and instability. Look for skin perforation (open fracture, grade 1) and examine the distal status regarding circulation and nerve function. X-ray the entire tibia. Occasionally there is a need for supplementary bone isotope scanning or MRI.

*Treatment.* Primary rough reduction of the fracture, stabilise temporarily with splinting, plaster-of-cast splint or vacuum cushions. Cover wounds as sterile as possible.
   Non-displaced fractures (or <1 cm shortening) can be treated with rotational-stable full leg plaster-of-cast (from the groin to the toes) for the first 2–4 weeks and then (when the fracture has begun to "stiffen") a lower leg cast, PTB-cast or orthosis followed by gradually increased weight bearing; the grade is determined by the fracture type. X-ray check-up after 7–10 days. Normal healing time 8–12 weeks. Children are as a rule treated the entire period of 6–10 weeks with full leg cast.

S.-A. Sölveborn, *Emergency Orthopedics*,
DOI 10.1007/978-3-642-41854-9_10, © Springer-Verlag Berlin Heidelberg 2014

Displaced (closed) lower leg fractures are reduced in general anaesthesia and, if a good position is achieved, continuous treatment as for an insignificantly displaced fracture mentioned above. In other cases nonemergency surgery is performed as long as the swelling is not too extensive and if the distal status is okay after having applied a strict elevation and an elastic bandage under a possible cast splint. Diaphyseal tibial fractures will most often be operated on with an intramedullary nail and locking screws. Comminute (and often open) fractures are treated with external fixation using a simple, double or so-called hybrid frame. Open fractures require antibiotic therapy and tetanus prophylaxis after wound culture and wound revision is completed.

*Isolated fibular fracture* S82.4 (most often proximally situated) usually occurs by direct trauma or an ankle injury with syndesmosis rupture (so-called C-type) at the same time and needs as a rule only unloading until the patient is pain free, but with greater displacement surgery has to be performed to avoid pseudoarthrosis development.

## Gastrocnemius Rupture ("Tennis Leg") * S86.1

*Diagnosis.* A distension injury involving a rupture in the muscle–tendon junction (MTJ) distally in the medial gastrocnemius belly (see Fig. 1). Sudden pain typically with motion exercise, sports or playing makes tiptoeing unable. Fairly often middle-aged persons. Tenderness in the rupture area with an initially palpable defect in the muscle–tendon region then swelling due to bleeding and oedema.

*Treatment.* Customary treatment of soft tissue injury including compression bandaging, elevation, initial non-weight bearing and unloaded motion, but from day 3–5 cautious strength and flexibility training. It can take 6–12 weeks to fully recover.

## Achilles Tendon Rupture * S86.0

*Diagnosis.* Most often in sports (59 % and then mostly in recreational exercise – 75–85 %, most common in badminton, 40–45 %), men highly overrepresented, ratio 2:1–12:1 to women and more among "white collar professions". Remarkably invariable average age about 35–40 years, most often on the left side (60 %). Very seldom heel tendon problems before the rupture (10–20 %), thus most often "like a bolt from the blue".

Sudden pain, which relatively soon rescinds. The patient, and also the surrounding persons, often experiences an audible snap and consequently turns around to see who gave a kick from behind to the leg of the patient! Difficulties in weight bearing, cannot do foot lift off properly when walking, and cannot tiptoe. The plantar flexion capacity significantly decreased. However, be aware that the long flexors, the tibial

**Fig. 1** Rupture of the
muscle–tendon junction of
the medial gastrocnemius, a
so-called tennis leg

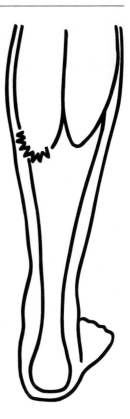

posterior and fibular/peroneal muscles also plantar flexion the foot. Palpation tenderness but seldom any great swelling. On the other hand an evident defect – a gap or sulcus in the tendon 2–5 cm from the calcaneal attachment. Positive (Doherty-)Thompson sign (or Simmonds sign) in 96 % of the cases, i.e. failure of plantar flexion of the foot when squeezing the calf musculature lying prone with freely hanging feet (see Fig. 2).

A simple clinical diagnosis – still 12–28 % of Achilles tendon ruptures (ATR) are reported to be missed at the acute examination! Ultrasound or MRI not necessary, but can assist the diagnosis.

**Fig. 2** Thomson's
(Simmonds') test with
squeezing around the calf: a
plantar flexion reaction
speaks against an Achilles
tendon rupture

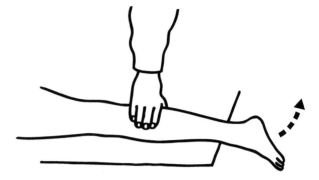

*Treatment.* Surgery with direct suture (can be done policlinically) is preferred, especially for younger patients (under 65 years) and patients with fairly high activity demands, including all athletes, when the rupture is close to the attachment on the calcaneus or when the tendon parts do not come into contact during plantar flexion of the foot. Postoperatively different approaches: an active model with a cast splint, in the attained ankle position during 2 weeks and this removed several times a day to allow cautious flexion–extension movement of the ankle, and after that use of a walker boot with gradually increasing weight bearing or a more passive model with a lower leg plaster-of-cast in pes-equino position for 3 weeks, then a heel-equipped plaster-of-cast allowing weight bearing up to full loading during an additional time of 3 weeks. A concept of early postoperative motion with a stirrup frame around a freely movable hanging foot can also be used; the frame is fixed to a PTB-lower leg cast, on which an immediate weight bearing is allowed.

Nonsurgical treatment (possible for elderly and persons with low function demands) uses a lower leg cast in pes-equino position for 3–4 weeks, then renewed cast in plantigrade position (right angle) with start of weight bearing at the end of a new 4 week period.

There is also a functional nonsurgical treatment with orthosis, which gradually is reset with diminishing pes-equino positions.

## Partial Achilles Tendon Rupture

Most often only slight pain initially, deterioration upon weight bearing. A distinctly tender point can be palpated and swelling occurs (palpate with thumb – index finger grip on both sides of the tendon simultaneously). Is treated with "active rest" for 2–4 weeks, possibly anti-inflammatory medication for 3 days and perhaps shoe heel heightening for some few weeks.

## Tibialis Anterior Tendon Rupture (traumatic) S86.2

*Diagnosis.* Almost always penetrative injury with a cut wound. Weak active dorsal extension of the foot.

*Treatment.* Surgery with exploration, wound revision, tendon suture and plaster-of-cast splint.

# Lower Leg Pain

## Acute Compartment Syndrome * T79.6

*Diagnosis.* Increased pressure in one or some of the four undistendable fascia rooms of the lower leg: anterior, lateral, posterior deep and posterior superficial, leading to ischemia, diminished arteriovenous pressure difference and decreased microcirculation in connection with fractures or contusions, chiefly in the lower leg, but can also develop in the forearm, the hand, the anterior thigh and the foot. Oedema and venous congestion deteriorate the condition in a vicious circle, and already after a few (4–5) hours the muscles and nerve tissues could suffer irreversible injuries and become necrotic!

Disproportionately severe pain in relation to the injury or surgical procedure, which is deteriorated by passive stretching of the muscles in question, swelling with a very tense, almost wooden hard, tender musculature with reduced function. Somewhat later in the process paraesthesia and impaired sensibility, but distal circulation can be normal with palpable peripheral pulses, since the tissue pressure seldom exceeds the arterial pressure, and the capillary circulation in the toes (and the fingers, respectively) is in general normal.

*Treatment.* Intramuscular pressure measurement resulting in 40 mmHg or a difference to the diastolic blood pressure <30 mmHg is an indication for acute fasciotomy (the normal intramuscular pressure is around 5–10 mmHg). Cut the plaster-of-cast and loosen the bandages. Keep the body part on heart level. Adjust analgesics so as not to disguise clinical signs. No ice or cold pack application!

## Stress Fracture (Tibia, Fibula) * M84.3G

*Diagnosis.* Almost half of all stress fractures, insufficiency fractures, affect the lower leg, most often localised to the distal or proximal third parts transition zones

S.-A. Sölveborn, *Emergency Orthopedics*,
DOI 10.1007/978-3-642-41854-9_11, © Springer-Verlag Berlin Heidelberg 2014

to the middle third of the tibia and the distal part of fibula. Rapidly increased training intensity with heavy loading (hard surface and insufficient shock absorbing) is the most important trigger mechanism. Acute debut of intense local, almost pinpoint pain at weight bearing occurs most often in connection with longer training sessions, can disappear at rest but recurs at once with strenuous activity, with time also aching at rest. Be aware of the combination amenorrhea, stress fracture and anorexia in thin female athletes.

X-ray in the early phase is often negative, while callus formation can be seen after some weeks. Bone isotope scanning, scintimetry, positive 1–2 days after symptom start and MRI also secure the diagnosis early.

*Treatment.* Non-weight bearing with crutch sticks for 6–8 weeks for the tibia and 4 weeks for the fibula. "Alternative training" is advised, e.g. bicycling and wet-vest running in water. Then slow return to normal training.

A more severe, but rare, variant of tibial stress fracture with the appearance of a blow of an axe on the anterior cortical part of the middle tibia, has a bad prognosis with the risk of pseudoarthrosis development and can require surgical fixation, also relatively good results with shock wave therapy (ECSWT) for these.

## Medial Tibial (Stress) Syndrome (MTS, "Shin Splints") M76.8

*Diagnosis.* The most common overuse injury in athletes. Pain from the fascia on the medial border of the tibia, especially the distal 2/3. The pain gradually increases and the patient has to interrupt running. Most of these patients hyperpronate their feet or have externally rotated lower legs. Palpation tenderness along the medial tibial border, most often maximally about 10 cm from the medial malleolus. X-ray can show a diffuse thickening of the medial corticalis, and bone isotope scan shows a diffuse increased uptake along wide parts of the tibial border. Can sometimes be interpreted as a preliminary stage of stress fracture.

*Treatment.* Training adjustment with reduction of the dose, cautious alternative training, stretching of the lower leg muscles (also the calf – m. tibialis posterior has its attachment in the region) and individual orthotic insoles. In persistent cases day care surgery with fasciotomy and release along the medial tibial border can be performed with very good results.

## Muscle Hernia (Anterior) M62.8

*Diagnosis.* Painful swelling, often 2–4 cm in diameter at about the middle of the anterior compartment, deteriorated by strenuous activity. A palpable defect in the fascia and tenderness there, but the condition can also be pain free. Note the vicinity to n. fibularis/peroneus superficialis.

*Treatment.* No special acute action is needed more than an elastic bandage, but if persisting or accentuating pain, fasciotomy and/or fascioplasty (with care taken to the nerve) can be indicated.

## Fibular (Peroneal) Nerve Entrapment (Caput Fibulae) G57.3

*Diagnosis.* Pain, numbness and paraesthesia down the lateral side of the lower leg. Impaired sensitivity over the anterior compartment and tenderness on palpation of the posterior, lateral range of the collum next to the fibular head. Can have normal EMG. Differential diagnoses: Lumbar nerve root compression/disc hernia and proximal fibular fracture.

*Treatment.* Avoid pressure on the area, e.g. when sitting with crossed legs or in secretary position with the foot outstretched backwards. Neurolysis of the nervus fibularis communis can rather frequently be indicated.

## Lumbar Nerve Compression (Disc Hernia) * M54.3

*Diagnosis.* Peripheral neurological symptoms from the nerve roots in the corresponding nerve dermatomes in the lower leg, i.e. L4, L5 and S2, very little L3.

*Treatment.* See the chapter "Lumbar Back Pain".

## Achilles Tendalgia, Achilles (Paratendinosis) * M76.6

*Diagnosis.* Acute heel tendon pain can occur after a rapid increase of the effort dose and intensity, above all running on hard surfaces, improper shoes and foot malposition, especially hyperpronation are important contributing causes. A remarkably great proportion, however, begins without any known intensive mechanical loading. The condition can also be an acute exacerbation of a longer standing Achilles paratendinosis with, in the typical cases, a spool-shaped thickening, which in fact relatively seldom (20 %) is constituted of a partial rupture (in studied surgical patient groups). The inadequate term "Achilles tendinitis" has so far doubtfully also been used for such cases with longer duration, but after the earliest phase of a limited number of days, there is no "inflammation" in or around the tendon, proven by histology, gene technology and microdialysis.

Local swelling, tenderness (especially from lateral thumb-index finger squeezing) and possibly squeaking/crepitus can be felt over the heel tendon, where redness also can occur very early in the course.

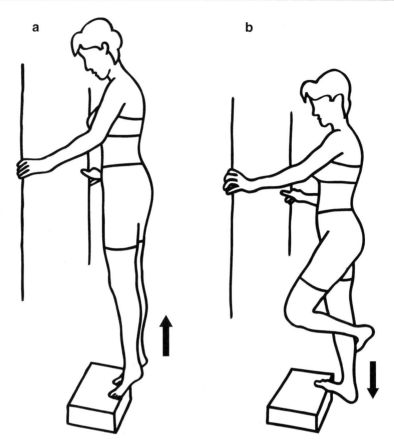

**Fig. 1** Eccentric Achilles tendon training, while standing, e.g. on a step of a staircase reach a heel-raising position with both feet (the other (healthy) foot is used for assistance), then drop the affected heel downwards with full weight of the body (15 × 3 × II for 3 months)

*Treatment.* Activity modification – training adjustment with active rest! Cold therapy and anti-inflammatory medication for a short period (up to 10–15 days), but local cortisone injection should *not* be given (due to inhibition of the fibroblasts and the collagen degrading effect). If crepitus is felt, intravenous anticoagulant therapy is administrated, heparin 15,000 IU × 1, repeat after one day and possibly after an additional day, depending on the symptom response. Individual foot orthotics is fitted. If there is remaining pain, referral to physiotherapist for eccentric calf muscle training (see Fig. 1) for 3 months with 15 repetitions in three sets twice daily with flexed and straight knee, respectively, under certain pain reaction, calf/Achilles tendon stretching, preferably with the PNF-method (contract-relax-stretch technique; see Fig. 3 of chapter "Foot Pain", page 28). Avoid heightening shoe heels, which in the long-term perspective make the situation worse with shortening of the Achilles tendon. Surgery (exploration with tenolysis) can be indicated when conservative therapy is futile after 3 months.

# Deep Venous Thrombosis (DVT) * I80.3

*Diagnosis.* Swelling of the calf or the entire lower leg with discomfort and tenderness on palpation or squeezing, there can be venous dilatation but also feeling of cold. Positive Homan sign, i.e. pain on passive dorsal extension of the ankle, but this is not a completely reliable test for thrombosis. Risk factors are, e.g. age over 40 years, heredity, immobilization or paresis, previous DVT, cancer, obesity, varicose veins, congestive heart failure, myocardial infarction, stroke, high-dose oestrogen medication and fractures of the pelvis, hip or leg. Verified by ultrasound scanning or venography.

*Treatment.* Anticoagulant therapy in an internal medicine department.

# Superficial Thrombophlebitis I80.0

*Diagnosis.* Redness and warmth with swelling and tenderness, most often in tissue with varicose veins.

*Treatment.* Hirudoid ointment with a 10–15 cm length applied twice daily.

# Part V

# Knee

# Knee Injuries

*General aspects of and important advice for knee disorders:*

*Pay attention to the most common significant knee injury, namely, O'Donoghue's classic unhappy triad (MCL + medial meniscus + ACL) and the fact that* **haemarthrosis** *(especially if appearing rapidly) should be considered as an anterior cruciate ligament rupture, until proven otherwise (ACL is injured in 60–80 % of cases). Observe that all swollen knees should be* **punctured** *and* **aspirated** *(for diagnosis, symptom relief and counteraction of the quadriceps inhibition). All patients with knee problems should be instructed to perform* **quadriceps exercises** *(see Fig. 1)! Be observant of the fact that knee pain (especially anterio-medial localisation) could be referred pain from a* **hip fracture**! *Always perform a knee stability examination (media-lateral and anterio-posterior, respectively) with the knee in slight flexion (20–30°).*

---

## Trauma

### Contusion S80.0

*Diagnosis.* Direct trauma, giving pain locally and swelling with bleeding, can hit blood vessels in the synovium and result in degree of haemarthrosis without any other significant injury, such as ligament rupture. X-ray should be taken.

*Treatment.* Elastic bandage, quadriceps muscle training (see Fig. 1) at once, weight bearing at a tolerable level.

### Collateral Ligament Rupture * S83.4

*Diagnosis.* The most common knee injury; medial ligament ruptures are included in 40 % of all knee injuries. Most often trauma from the side with the knee in slight

S.-A. Sölveborn, *Emergency Orthopedics*,
DOI 10.1007/978-3-642-41854-9_12, © Springer-Verlag Berlin Heidelberg 2014

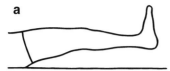 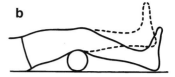

**Fig. 1** Quadriceps muscle training: (**a**) Isometrically elevating the leg 20–30 cm for up to 20 s, e.g. by sitting on a bed with support from the arms behind the back; should be repeated at least two to three times. (**b**) Dynamically training by full extension exercises from a knee joint angle of about 30° with a support, such as a cylindrical cushion or a small pile of books with towels around, etc., under the hollow of the knee; preferably repeated at least 40 times and for two to three sets

flexion; valgus trauma causes medial collateral injury (MCL). Lateral ligament injury (LCL) is rare, a little more complicated and extra-articularly situated. The medial ligament is connected with the medial meniscus (not the case on the lateral side), which should be observed at the examination. Thus, a stable knee producing pain in valgus stress provocation can suggest a medial meniscus rupture or, of course, a partial ligament rupture. Observe that the varus–valgus stability must be tested with the knee in 20–30° of flexion; in full extension the posterior capsule is sufficiently stiff to give good stability. If laxity is observed in full extension, there is a severe injury, with the posterior capsule ruptured and, very likely also, a tear in the anterior cruciate ligament.

Pain will correspond to the extension of the ligament, but the joint as such will not be swollen in an isolated injury; however, there is still a restricted range-of-motion. Can be the initial phase of one of the most important common knee injury that people come to a emergency unit for, namely, *O'Donoghue's classic unhappy triad* with in consecutive order: MCL, medial meniscus and anterior cruciate ligament ruptures (S83.7) caused by valgus trauma in combination with external rotation of the lower leg (e.g. a ski sliding outwards or a football player that gets stuck with his boot in the pitch while being tackled by an opponent). Observe also the existence of the "pain paradox": a partial rupture often results in more pain than a total rupture.

*Treatment.* Good prognosis with nonoperative treatment, use a sideways stabilising articulated knee orthosis (e.g. of the type Genu Syncron), quadriceps training (see Fig. 1, above) immediately (physiotherapy can then be started after 2–3 days) and an elastic bandage underneath the orthosis; for moderate injuries sideward taping of the knee can also be performed. Controlled weight bearing is allowed, possibly crutch sticks for partial support for a short period of time. A plaster-of-cast or surgery for an isolated collateral ligament injury is contraproductive, as it will only extend the healing time.

## Meniscal Tear * S83.2, M23.2

*Diagnosis.* Rotational trauma to the knee, often in combination with flexion and, if there is additional external rotation, as the second step in the classic unhappy triad (see section "Collateral Ligament Rupture" above).

Pain and tenderness on palpation over the joint line – however, observe that also there is some tenderness over the medial (but not lateral!) joint space of a healthy knee (so compare with the contralateral side)! Sometimes joint effusion (see Fig. 2), but it will arise slowly and most often later in the course of events. Often a defect in extension ability that could stem from a mechanical locking of a displaced meniscal rupture, where the "bucket handle tear" is the most common. This has a vertical–longitudinal rupture, where the inner part (the bucket handle) is displaced into the joint compartment towards the intercondylar space. The extension defect could also be a pain-evoked muscle defence or due to an anterior cruciate ligament injury. The medial meniscus is injured five times more often than the lateral. A certain age variation exists so that younger individuals (often in sports) get central vertical and longitudinal ruptures, while older persons suffer degenerative frayed flap tears in or near the posterior part (the posterior "horn"). This flap tear is surprisingly common in the latter age group (in the sixth decade of life).

Positive McMurray and 1st Steinmann tests (the latter performed in fixed 90° of flexion and seems even more discriminative, especially for acute cases) with pain (and sometimes clicking or "popping") medially on external rotation and laterally on internal rotation of the lower leg and foot for medial and lateral meniscal tear, respectively.

*Treatment.* If effusion has occurred, knee joint puncture and aspiration is performed (see Fig. 3); no blood if isolated meniscal injury, can however be "raspberry juice coloured". If there is an extension defect ("locking") >15–20° with typical springy elastic resistance in the end position, revisit to a knee clinic very soon, as well as, when the patient is hard to examine due to pain reaction, preferably within 3–5 days in the latter situation to ensure a safe diagnosis. Quadriceps training (see Fig. 1, page 66), elastic bandage, consider crutch sticks for pain relief and referral to a physiotherapist. If there is a remaining extension

**Fig. 2** Examination of joint effusion, hydrops (a "bulge test"): Move the hand over the distal thigh from a level corresponding to the suprapatellar pouch milking the joint fluid downwards to the central knee area. Excessive joint fluid will be felt as a fluctuation on both sides of the patella and seen as a bulge

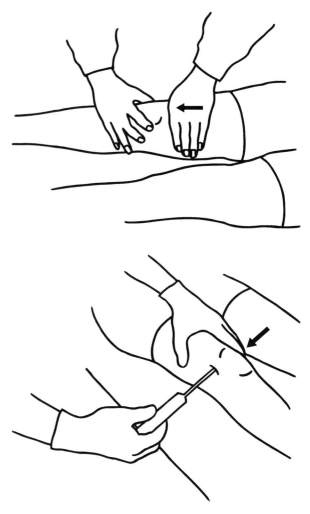

**Fig. 3** Knee joint aspiration from the lateral side, which may be made easier by a certain angulation pressure to the patella medially and insertion of the needle at the upper lateral patellar border

defect: arthroscopy within 2 weeks, this gives the possibility of performing a successful suture/fixation of the meniscal rupture or a partial resection. However, most patients with clinical signs of meniscal tear will in fact recover without surgery.

## Anterior Cruciate Ligament Tear * S83.5, M23.5

*Diagnosis.* Most often rotational trauma in sports, especially with valgus and external rotation of the lower leg as step 3 in the *classic unhappy triad* (see sections "Collateral Ligament Rupture" and "Meniscal Tear" above), and is in fact the most common significant knee injury and surely, without doubt, under diagnosed. About

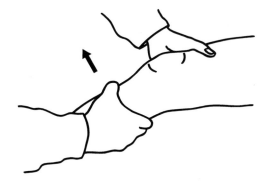

**Fig. 4** Lachman's test for sagittal laxity. With a stable grip around the distal thigh, the proximal lower leg is grasped and the tibia pulled forward with the knee at about 20° of flexion

75 % of anterior cruciate ligament injuries have concomitant meniscal tears. Female elite players in Olympic handball (and football) have four times more often injuries to the anterior cruciate ligaments (ACL) than their male equivalents. Most often a total rupture which results in rapid swelling (see Fig. 2, page 68) due to bleeding, thus a *haemarthrosis*, in 60–80 % of knee injuries this is caused by an ACL-rupture. A swelling within 30 min after a knee trauma should be considered an ACL-tear until the opposite has been proven. The patient also often feels as though something is broken in the knee, there is severe pain (often located centrally in the knee on a level just inferior to the apex patellae and pain also inwards from both anterio-medial and anterior-lateral direction) and a feeling as though the knee is going to dislocate. It can also be experienced as "giving way" when loading the knee after the injury. The Lachman's test (see Fig. 4), which is performed in about 20° of flexion, is positive with >90% certainty, while so-called anterior drawer test in 90° of flexion is a very unreliable method with false-negative outcomes in more than half of arthroscopically verified ruptures, and should thus be avoided, in order not to be deceived by the finding! Sagittal laxity can be hard to demonstrate if the patient has so much pain that muscle defence with contraction of the hamstring muscles occurs and stabilises the knee, since they attach below the knee joint. See the patient again after a few days for a new examination if it is difficult to perform a proper one in the acute phase. The diagnosis is clinical (and can even be made on telephone, provided that the given initial information in patient's history is correct!).

*Treatment.* Swelling should lead to knee puncture and aspiration (see Fig. 3; observe that an ACL-rupture can be present without swelling; furthermore, some-times a so-called swelling paradox can occur, i.e. the worst knee ligament injuries have no swelling at all, since a capsule tear also entails a sinking of the joint effusion down into the lower leg). Elastic bandage, knee muscle training and referral to a physiotherapist. Initially handle crutches to allow walking with almost no weight bearing, only footstep marking. No need for emergency surgery apart from exceptional cases. Always refer to a "knee orthopaedic surgeon" for follow-up with physical exam including pivot shift test (see Fig. 5) and decision

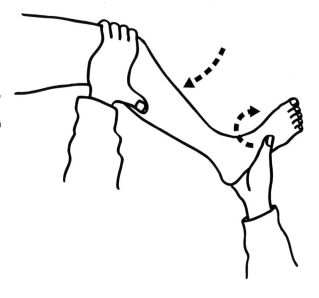

**Fig. 5** Pivot shift test, according to Macintosh, for anterior cruciate ligament insufficiency: Fully extended and the knee internally rotated with a valgus force applied, the knee is cautiously flexed and for a positive sign there is a "jerk" and/or a pain reaction at 20–40° (= subluxation of the lateral tibia condyle)

about arthroscopy. Before surgery with anterior cruciate ligament reconstruction is considered, an ACL-rehabilitation programme, including daily home exercises, should be performed for at least 3 months.

Advise the patient about avoiding "cutting sports", i.e. activities with sudden stops and twisting movements and to start immediately with thigh muscle exercises, especially strength exercises for the posterior part (hamstrings), as well as balance training such as one-leg standing with progressive difficulty from plane surface to wobble board; bicycle training 20 min daily can also be recommended. Knee bandage for the stimulation of proprioception, i.e. reflex mediated stabilisation. Mechanically, the knee cannot be stabilised to a sufficient extent with an orthosis.

## Eminentia Fracture S82.1, S83.5

*Diagnosis.* "The anterior cruciate ligament rupture of the child", where there is an avulsion fracture on the eminentia intercondylare tibiae, since the bone insertion is relatively weaker than the cruciate ligament itself, most common in the ages 8–13 years. Fairly severe pain, often an extension defect and acute effusion with haemarthrosis. Lachman's test positive. The X-ray shows the fracture, most evident on the side-to-side/lateral projection.

*Treatment.* Substantially displaced eminentia (grade 2 injury, 5 mm superiorly dislocated anterior edge) is treated surgically (within 10 days), and a grade 3 injury with completely loosened eminentia should be fixed and stabilised very soon; nowadays this can be performed using an arthroscopic technique. Other cases should be treated with knee puncture and aspiration alone. A cast is then applied in a hyperextended position and worn for 4–5 weeks, with weight bearing allowed.

## Posterior Cruciate Ligament Rupture S83.5

*Diagnosis.* Uncommon injury, most often in adolescents, more common in men than women. Most often powerful flexion violence or "dash-board injury" that hits the proximal lower leg from the anterior. Also from hyperextension trauma. Half of all injures occur in sports, half in traffic accidents and more than half of all have combination injuries. The posterior cruciate ligament (PCL) is injured only 1/10 as often as the anterior. The PCL is partly situated extra-articularly, probably the reason for the haemarthrosis with swelling not coming so fast, instead an effusion can appear gradually. Often severe pain, the diagnosis is clinical with posterior laxity, which also can be seen as a "hammock" sign, when the proximal tibia is translated posteriorly in 70–90° of flexion compared with the uninjured knee side by side (= "sag sign") or recurvatum position in full extension. Look for associated injuries in the knee.

*Treatment.* Customary elastic bandaging and quadriceps training (see Fig. 1, page 66) are particularly important, weight bearing as tolerated. Emergency surgery is not indicated, with an isolated PCL injury the prognosis is generally favourable, active rehabilitation training with physiotherapy.

## Patellar Dislocation S83.0

*Diagnosis.* Relatively severe direct or indirect trauma to the knee, often with torsion. Practically always lateral dislocation. More common in predisposed persons with increased joint laxity, patella alta and shallow sulcus or wide Q-angle (>20° for women and >15° for men). The patellar dislocation is usually reduced before the arrival at the emergency room. Often remaining haemarthrosis and medial patellar border tenderness on palpation (medial capsular rupture). Can have bone fragments from the medial edge of the patella or lateral femur condyle, but also big and/or multiple cartilage fragments, which are invisible on X-ray.

*Treatment.* Careful knee extension after pain relief, light pressure against the lateral part of the patella. Knee puncture and joint aspiration (see Fig. 3, page 68 and Fig. 6, page 72) if there is an effusion with haemarthrosis. If significant bone fragment: Surgery with arthroscopy and extraction or refixation.
Quadriceps training (see Fig. 1, page 66), referral to physiotherapist. If necessary locked orthosis/splint for about a week. A checkup is necessary due to the risk of

**Fig. 6** Knee puncture –
according to all the
recognized rules – using
sterile gloves, fenestrated
drape and hair protection; see
also the chapter "Basic
Injection Techniques"

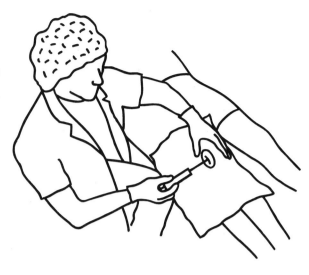

bone fragment, and if so, arthroscopy is indicated. *Recurrent dislocations:* Return visit to consider surgery, e.g. lateral release and later medial transposition of the tuberositas tibiae or sulcus reconstruction.

## Patellar Fracture S82.0

*Diagnosis.* Most often direct trauma, e.g. caused by a fall in elderly persons or somersault in younger persons, and the fracture can then be comminuted. Sometimes powerful distraction trauma that can result in a transverse fracture.

Tenderness on palpation and a diastasis if the fracture is displaced transversely, swelling and commonly haemarthrosis. Patients are frequently not able to raise the leg with a straight knee. Ordinary X-ray is sufficient.

*Treatment.* Joint puncture and evacuation of the haemarthrosis if evident effusion. An undisplaced longitudinal fracture does not need to be immobilised, instead the patient can be supplied with elastic bandage and handle crutches. Undisplaced transverse fractures can be treated with plaster-of-cast, but a knee orthosis of the type Genu Syncron with adjustable flexion position is still better. Start with a straight knee, gradually increasing flexion setting during 3–4 weeks. Weight bearing with straight knee is allowed from the beginning.

Displaced fractures are treated surgically, at least if the separation is >3–4 mm. If there is less dislocation, a knee plaster or an orthosis can be used for 6 weeks. Standard X-ray control after 7–10 days for all of the fracture types above. The most common surgical technique is circular cerclage and Kirschner pins, at times screw fixation. A stable osteosynthesis does not require plaster-of-cast postoperatively, and motion exercises can be started at once, as well as quadriceps muscle training (see Fig. 1, page 66).

## Femoral Condyle Fracture * S72.4

*Diagnosis.* Distal femoral fractures are most common in osteoporotic elderly with a fall, while often caused by heavy trauma in younger persons, mostly traffic accidents. Can extend supracondylarly and can then have a T- or Y-shape. Often intra-articular involvement, with effusion and haemarthrosis (with lots of "fat pearls" in the aspirated fluid). Can also result in injuries to nerves and blood vessels – perform a distal status examination! Plain X-ray gives the diagnosis; instability/ laxity and local tenderness is virtually always present.

*Treatment.* Knee joint puncture (see Fig. 3, page 68) and evacuation of the haemarthrosis. Primary stabilisation with a plaster splint, then surgery with osteosynthesis so that joint congruence and stability are attained. Consider just using plaster-of-cast or orthosis when the joint surfaces are essentially intact or if the patient is a bad object for surgery in those cases: repeat X-ray controls of the fracture position. Treatment of osteoporosis, see the chapter "Osteoporosis".
**Epiphyseolysis fracture** in children, usually after a valgus or a hyperextension trauma, is treated with a knee plaster-of-cast if undisplaced, while a displaced one is reduced (closed) in general anaesthesia; for sufficient stability, fixation with crossed pins over the physis is sometimes required. Screw fixation parallel to the physis is used more seldom. Postoperatively plaster-of-cast for 4 weeks. In children younger than 10 years a malposition of 10–20° in the frontal plane can be accepted. Check after a week with X-ray.

## Tibial Condyle (Plateau) Fracture * S82.1

*Diagnosis.* Most common in elderly with osteoporosis and indirect varus or valgus trauma. Most often the lateral tibia condyle is involved in a shear split fracture, but more commonly a comminuted compression fracture resulting in an incongruent cut in the articular surface. Usually caused by violent trauma in younger persons and the fracture can then include both condyles. Always haemarthrosis with "fat pearls" in the aspirated fluid, tenderness and pain with movement and often latero-medial laxity. After plain X-ray, tomography has to be done to map the fracture system.

*Treatment.* Knee joint puncture (see Fig. 3, page 68) with evacuation of the haemarthrosis. If stable in valgus–varus provocation, and <2 (–4) mm of depression without a considerable posterior compression, an articulated orthosis can be fitted to the knee after an elastic bandage has been applied underneath. Non-weight bearing. Arrange for a check-up after 1 week, this should include an X-ray. Consider a plaster-of-cast of a sawed lid-and-chest type, allowing daily uplifting of the leg for movement exercises, suitable for certain well-cooperative patients. If unstable knee and displaced fracture, surgery with reduction and osteosynthesis, so that the fracture preferably will be stable for training; postoperatively the use of a CPM (continuous passive motion)-machine can be beneficial. Elevation, mobilisation and cautious walking by just marking the steps initially; full weight bearing can generally be started after 3 months. Observe the cases caused by osteoporosis; see the chapter "Osteoporosis" for what measures to take.

## Knee Dislocation S83.1

*Diagnosis.* Rare, but can be caused by knee trauma with very heavy forces, e.g. motor bike accidents or fall in a ski jump. Is defined as ruptures of at least three of the four main ligaments (MCL, LCL, ACL and PCL), corresponding laxity in at least three directions. Considerable risk of vascular (a. poplitea) and nerve injuries, perform distal status examination! Every third patient has neurological deficit in the area supplied by n. fibularis/peroneus, and 10 % have an arterial injury. If dislocation: Reduce of course immediately! X-ray and order a MRT or angiography.

*Treatment.* If any vascular injury, immediate surgery (if delay >8 h: 80 % risk of amputation), while the ligament injuries can be taken care of later (after some weeks). An elastic bandage is used initially and an orthosis or a cast splint.

## Referred Pain from Hip Fracture * S72.0/S72.1

*Diagnosis.* It is important to be aware that knee pain, especially if located anterio-medially (somewhat extended), can be due to a hip fracture, which, e.g. can occur in an elderly patient without significant trauma, in fact almost spontaneously upon weight bearing, without the patient feeling any pain in the hip region from the beginning! In the knee exam, a (rotation) test of the hip should therefore always be included, especially in the elderly. Internal rotation in the end position is typically the most sensitive for pain in the hip joint (see Fig. 1 of chapter "Thigh and Groin Pain", page 98). Moreover, see section "Cervical, Trochanteric or Subtrochanteric Hip Fracture" in the chapter "Hip and Pelvis Injuries".

# Overload

## Patellar Tendon Rupture S83.6

*Diagnosis.* After a sudden or forceful load on the extensor apparatus in younger persons, often male athletes, but also in elderly, caused by a quite modest loading in usually poorly active individuals. Sometimes predisposing factors like diabetes, RA and other systemic inflammatory conditions. Local pain and swelling. Can be a partial rupture, when the patient manages to extend the knee, but the strength is always reduced. Often a palpable defect if the disruption is considerably large. Patients often report having heard or experienced an audible snap, like that of a broken rubber band. Clinical diagnosis, ultrasound can verify. X-ray can show a proximally situated patella.

*Treatment* of choice is almost always surgery with tendon repair and fixation.

## Quadriceps Tendon Rupture S76.1

*Diagnosis.* The counterpart just proximally to the patella tendon ruptures (see above) when a heavy loading is put on the extensor apparatus, most common in elderly or middle-aged men. A palpable defect, most often centrally, proximal to the patella, inability or substantial weakness when attempting to extend the knee against resistance. Haemarthrosis, X-ray can show a more distally located patella (patella baja) and avulsed fragment(s) of bone corresponding to the tendon insertion. Ultrasound can confirm the rupture.

*Treatment.* Surgery with tendon repair, osteosuture if the disruption is close to the patella.

## Jumper's Knee M76.5

*Diagnosis.* Insertalgia at the attachment of the patellar tendon on the apex of the patella, most often caused by a partial rupture located proximally in the patellar tendon "underneath"/posteriorly (se Fig. 7). Common in sports, the prevalence in, e.g. volleyball is 40 %, also occurs in football (soccer). Often presents after sudden loading, such as the eccentric moment involved in landing after a jump; this is followed by a pain attack, but there can also be a gradual onset of pain. Tenderness on palpation over the apex patellae, especially at "apicitis test", when the inferior pole of the patella is angled forward through pressure downwards and distally against the proximal border of the patella, "Puddu sign". Often pain as from

**Fig. 7** Jumper's knee with changes caused by a partial rupture in depth at the proximal attachment of the patellar tendon

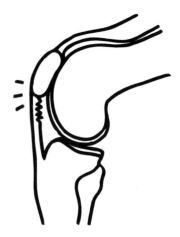

patellalgia, PFPS, with cinema/movie sign, knee pain when walking downwards in stairs or a hill slope etc., is reported.

*Treatment.* Training adjustment, patella strap bandage circularly over the patellar tendon and stretching of the quadriceps daily. Some patients experience good results with eccentric strength training. Local injection of corticosteroids (mixed with local anaesthetics) can have a good effect if given in under and up against the patellar tendon insertion. Notably many patients continue to day surgery, where excision of the altered tendon tissue is done, and detachment of fibrous adherences, that almost always exist to the underlying synovial Hoffa fat pad and thereby produce impingement-resembling pain on pressure and squeezing.

## Meniscus Tear * S83.2, M23.2

See in the section "Trauma" above.

## Mb Osgood–Schlatter M92.5A

*Diagnosis.* Loading correlated "apophysitis" on the tuberositas tibiae, almost only in older children and young adults, especially in the middle of the growth spurt (12–18 years), more common in boys ("errand boy disease") and often bilateral (certain heredity). Is noted to occur particularly in sports with lots of jump and hop training or in football. Traction disturbance in the growth zone. Tenderness on palpation over the bulging enlargement on the tibial tubercle, where the patellar tendon is attached. Can even lead to an isolated ossicle or free projected sequestre on X-ray in the tuberositas area. Pain on exertion of the extensor apparatus and in kneeling activities. X-ray in straight-forward cases is unnecessary.

*Treatment.* Training adjustment with dose reduction, well-balanced activity, quadriceps training (see Fig. 1, page 66) with strength exercises and stretching. Strict activity restriction is not necessary in the children. Self-marking condition for tolerable exercise. The prognosis is good for almost all. Occasionally long-lasting function-limiting problems with a loose sequester (or ossifications) that can be an indication for surgical extraction.

## Mb Sinding–Larsen/Sven Johansson Disease M92.4

*Diagnosis.* The equivalent to Mb Schlatter but at the proximal patellar tendon insertion, apex patellae, which is tender on palpation. Pain when loading the extensor apparatus. Most often seen in physically active boys.

*Treatment.* As for Mb Schlatter (see above), also patella strap bandage, as for jumper's knee, can be tried. The condition most often disappears spontaneously in ½–1 year.

## Overuse

## Patellalgia/Patellofemoral Arthralgia (PFA, PFPS) * M22.2

*Diagnosis.* The most common clinical knee pain syndrome, traditionally, but incorrectly and misleadingly, called "chondromalacia patellae"; cartilage alterations are, however, seldom present. Anterior knee pain (often bilateral) around and just inferior to the patella. Onset is usually insidious and spontaneous, but can also occur after direct trauma. Worsened by activity, becomes evident in, e.g. sports. Shows cinema/movie sign, i.e. pain on sitting with 90° of knee flexion for a longer time. Aggravated by walking in stairs, more downwards than upwards, downhill walking or running with eccentric loading. Joint effusion is uncommon, but many patients report a buckling and cushion-like feeling in the knee. Weakness, as though the knee were about to give way of muscle reflex type. Typical sudden pain attacks from synovial impingement. The patient comes to the clinic due to the worsening synovitis. May have "inward-looking" patellae pointing towards each other (a sign of internal femoral torsion), foot hyperpronation and genu recurvatum, hypotrophy and weakness in the vastus medialis muscle. Tenderness on palpation around the patella border, most typically at the medial–distal corner. Positive Clarke's sign, i.e. pain on quadriceps contraction with the hand as light pressure against the proximal patella pole, positive compression test according to Cleveland. Apprehension sign positive with pain when the patella is pushed laterally over the femur condyle (during simultaneous flexion from extended position; see Fig. 8). Often stiffness in the quadriceps muscle (tested in a prone position), but also restricted flexibility in the hamstrings. Commonly, lateralization of the patella on quadriceps contraction can be demonstrated by the "Sölveborn pen test", where a

**Fig. 8** Apprehension sign, a
provocation test of patellalgia
with concomitant lateral
laxity: The patella is pushed
in lateral direction during
simultaneous flexion from an
extended knee position

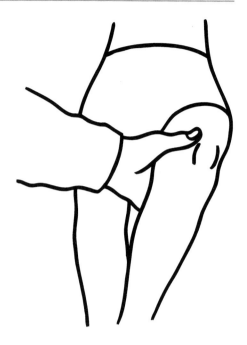

pen is put at the centre of patella, whose movement on active quadriceps contraction (start of straight leg raising) is illustrated by the direction and length of the formed ink line. Often increased Q-angle (>20–22° in women and >15–18° in men).

*Treatment.* Quadriceps strength training, isometrically and dynamically (see Fig. 1, page 66), especially for m. vastus medialis (obliquus). Stretching of the quadriceps, hamstrings and tractus iliotibialis (see Fig. 9). Referral to a physiotherapist. A certain amount of pain during exercise therapy is allowed, up to 20 on a 100 graded scale in order not to lose tempo and strength during the rehabilitation. Patella stabilising orthosis with a lateral pelot and customised foot orthotics are very often advisable. Medial patella taping according to Jenny McConnell. Training adjustment and control after a rehabilitation period of 2–3 months for judgement to surgery, e.g. lateral release.

**Fig. 9** Stretching of the fascia lata/tractus iliotibialis: With support from the hand of the same side as the stretched leg – against a low table or equivalent – let the hip sink down (by a slight lateral movement) so that the body forms a "C", and hold the position (the stretch may be accentuated by moving the pelvis a little backwards)

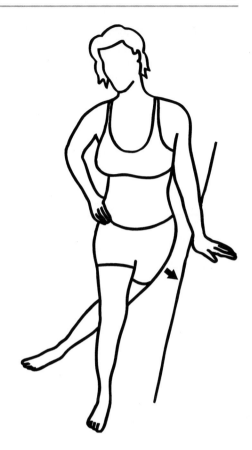

## Synovial Impingement * M65.9G

See the chapter "Knee Pain".


## Loose Body with Knee Locking M23.4

*Diagnosis.* Acute mechanical knee locking, i.e. extension defect when the loose body gets stuck, wedging itself in the joint space. Simultaneous pain reaction can occur due to synovial swelling with impingement phenomena. Loose fragments can emanate from *osteochondrosis dissecans, meniscal tear, osteoarthrosis, patella dislocation and cruciate ligament injury.* If a loose body stays in the fossa intercondylaris (the "notch"), it does not necessarily have to cause problems (can sometimes be "shafted" with a fibrous synovial band). X-ray can reveal an osteochondrosis defect and a bone-dense body (which does not need to be "free" and loose in the joint, but can adhere to the capsule – take a tunnel or a notch radiograph projection) and MRT meniscal and cartilage injuries.

*Treatment.* Arthroscopic extraction and treatment for the original lesion. Consider refixation in cases of fresh detachment or larger bone–cartilage fragments.


## Prepatellar Bursitis ("Carpet Layer's, Housemaid's or Carpenter's Knee") M70.4

See the chapter "Knee Swelling".

# Knee Pain

*NB! Quadriceps muscle training* (see Fig. 1 of chapter "Knee Injuries", page 66) *with isometric and dynamic end extension exercises should generally be started at once for all knee disorders!*

## Patellalgia/Patellofemoral Arthralgia (PFA, PFPS) * M22.2

See the chapter "Knee Injuries".

## Patellar Instability (Subdislocations) M22.1

*Diagnosis.* Patellar instability (can be a second stage in a patellalgia development), see also section "Patellar Dislocation" in the chapter "Knee Injuries". Sudden pain attacks, feeling of patellar instability, can occur as a result of excess loading, including rotation or twisting, e.g. in sports or dance. Often central retro- and subpatellar pain with forward radiation anterio-medially. There can be an increased Q-angle and easily mobile patella (see Fig. 8 of chapter "Knee Injuries", page 78).

*Treatment.* Same as for *Patellalgia* and *Patellar dislocation*, quadriceps training (see Fig. 1 of chapter "Knee Injuries", page 66), patella stabilizing orthosis with lateral pelot can be attempted, stretching of the quadriceps, hamstrings and tractus IT and foot orthotics if there is a foot hyperpronation (to avoid rotational loading on the knee).

## Synovial Impingement * M65.9G

*Diagnosis.* Typically sudden pain attacks, which can also cause pain locking in the affected knee. The synovia is then swollen, bulging, sometimes lacerated (sea-grass

S.-A. Sölveborn, *Emergency Orthopedics*,
DOI 10.1007/978-3-642-41854-9_13, © Springer-Verlag Berlin Heidelberg 2014

or finger-like) pain sensitive synovial tissue being interponated and subject to squeezing. The synovial irritation can be a consequence of another knee disorder, such as meniscal or cruciate ligament injury, patellalgia (PFPS), osteoarthrosis (OA) or osteochondrosis. The synovium produces joint fluid, which leads to effusion, hydrops. Continuous pain at rest can also be present. Palpation tenderness most commonly occurs in the parapatellar synovial, mainly anterio-medial, area.

*Treatment.* Immediate quadriceps training (see Fig. 1 of chapter "Knee Injuries", page 66), elastic bandage (stimulating the proprioception) and treatment of the underlying disorder. Analgesics can be indicated, and an initial short cure of anti-inflammatory medication in order to alleviate the synovitis reaction can also be considered. Recurrent attacks can necessitate arthroscopy with synovial shaving when appropriate.

## Osteochondrosis (Dissecans, OCD) M93.2G

*Diagnosis.* A disorder that has been explained by reduced blood supply to a bone/ cartilage area, commonly (85 %) at the "inner" lateral part of the medial femur condyle and more often in boys. The affected area can be unstable and gradually loosen from its attachment, leading to pain (thus dominating medially) and aching after activity. In the final stage the "osteochondrite" will be released as a loose body, which can cause a mechanical locking with a consequential extension defect. Most patients are young, often under 16 years of age, but the disorder can also occur in somewhat older individuals, who then often can report previous long-standing minor symptoms, indicating an early first appearance. The patient's history does not usually include any trauma. Pain correlated to loading and swelling tendency. A plain X-ray is most often sufficient.

*Treatment.* Quadriceps training (see Fig. 1 of chapter "Knee Injuries", page 66), avoidance of the pain-provoking activity and quick follow-up visit with respect to extension defect. If problems persist, especially locking phenomena: arthroscopy to refix or extract the bone/cartilage fragment.

## Loose Body in the Joint M23.4

See the chapter "Knee Injuries".

## Osteoarthrosis (OA, "Osteoarthritis") * M17.1/M17.3

*Diagnosis.* On the whole, a mere half of the population with radiological signs of knee OA, in fact, has any knee pain! The correlation between the X-ray appearance and patient symptoms is weak or nonexistent. Arthrosis is not necessarily an inexorable, progressive disorder, but can develop in three directions: alleviation to symptom freedom ("aching out"), persisting symptoms with an often fluctuating, variable course or gradual deterioration. Observe that as high proportion as 60–90 % of patients with injured anterior cruciate ligaments will have signs of arthrosis on X-ray already 10–15 years after the trauma (which probably depends on the original impact trauma and not the laxity per se). The patient can present with heavy aching at rest, pain correlated with loading and knee swelling. Often sudden pain attacks from impingement of swollen, irritated synovia. Weakness with quadriceps inhibition due to effusion and pain. Crepitus in the joint, lockings and loose bodies can occur. Restricted range of motion is generally present and osteophytes along the joint edges can be palpated. Knee deformity and varus–valgus angling in the more advanced stages. X-ray should be taken in standing position with weight bearing.

*Treatment.* If effusion, knee puncture with aspiration (as always; see Fig. 3 of chapter "Knee Injuries", page 68), elastic bandage, instruction and demonstration of quadriceps training (see Fig. 1 of chapter "Knee Injuries", page 66). Knee training has scientifically been shown to be the most important factor for the result of the treatment. Exacerbation phases should be treated with a cure of an anti-inflammatory drug; stick crutches should be considered. Maintained but modified physical activity. Referral to a physiotherapist for strength and flexibility training with home exercises. Shoe orthotics or sole build-up with lateral (most commonly indicated) or medial wedge in order to direct the loading line towards the non-symptomatic side of the knee in case of unilateral osteoarthrosis. Follow-up to determine whether surgery, mainly arthroplasty, but also arthroscopic joint "toilet" with resection of bulging synovia, joint irrigation, extraction of loose bodies and resection of defect meniscus parts, can have good results. Advice on weight reduction is important – a decrease of only 5 kg (or 15 % of bodyweight in other studies) has been proven to give significant symptom reduction with pain relief.

## Arthritis of the Knee: Crystal Synovitis M11.9G, RA M05.8G/ M06.9G, Psoriatic M07.3G, Septic M00.0/M00.2/M00.9, Postinfectious M03.2 *

*Diagnosis.* Three basic categories of arthritis: *degenerative* (osteoarthrosis, OA, the most common form), *destructive* (autoimmune, inflammatory, RA, gout, psoriasis) and *secondary* (posttraumatic, instability related, septic). Highest priority to diagnose a bacterial arthritis, but luckily this form is rarer than what is commonly thought. It predominantly occurs postoperatively or post-traumatically after wound injuries. These aetiologies are followed by haematogenous spread in frequency. The knee joint is more often affected than other joints. Pyrophosphate arthritis is the most common arthritis in the elderly, more often women. Younger adults primarily suffer from reactive arthritis or RA.

The knee is warm (fever can occur with septic arthritis) and generally tender when touched, pain with movement both passively and actively and pain on weight bearing. Joint swelling restricts the range of motion, most evident in flexion, but also in extension; feeling of stiffness, popping and crepitus can occur.

*Treatment.* Knee puncture and aspiration (see Fig. 3 of chapter "Knee Injuries", page 68) if the joint fluid is muddy or cloudy, a microbiological culture and a direct microscopy are performed, additionally a crystal analysis and rinsing of the joint compartment with saline solution is also indicated. Bacterial arthritis as a rule has >50 white blood cells in the joint and the ratio glucose in the joint/blood less than 0.5. When infection is suspected, antibiotics are administered intravenously; cloxacillin is recommended in younger adults, or cephalosporins, which are the first choice in small children and elderly persons; this is followed by p.o ABX for 6 weeks. For other arthritis periodic medication with anti-inflammatory drugs can be given. Elastic bandaging and follow-up within 1–2 days if a septic aetiology is suspected, often admission to hospital and consideration of whether joint drainage or arthroscopy is indicated. However, repeated knee joint aspirations are also an adequate treatment regimen. Quadriceps training (see Fig. 1 of chapter "Knee Injuries", page 66) as usual for knee disorders; furthermore, therapy for the underlying cause.

## Baker's Cyst M71.2

*Diagnosis.* Swelling from a cyst in the fossa poplitea, a distended bursa (usually in the more medial area), often in connection to the joint space via a valve mechanism, but can also originate from the medial hamstring tendons. Often associated with an (sometimes asymptomatic) intra-articular disorder and simultaneous increased joint exudate and tenderness. Discomfort and a feeling of filling and stiffness in the posterior part of the knee, accentuated by squatting. Palpable non-pulsating swelling (differential diagnosis: arterial aneurysm!). The cyst can rupture acutely and produce swelling of the calf, imitating a deep venous thrombosis, or else leak slowly. The size of the cyst may often increase on knee activity and then decrease in rest. Ultrasound is indicated. Previously arthrography was performed for mapping, nowadays MRT.

*Treatment.* Primarily, treatment of the underlying intra-articular cause, e.g. meniscal tear (most often a degenerative posterior horn injury), osteoarthrosis (OA) and other causes of reactive synovitis. Knee puncture and aspiration if problems are severe. An arterial aneurysm has to be ruled out first. Surgical extirpation is seldom performed nowadays.

## Pes Anserine Insertalgia M70.5

*Diagnosis.* Pain in the area ("the goose foot") of the hamstrings attachment (semimembranosus, semitendinosus and gracilis) to the anterio-medial part of the medial tibia condyle with the underlying bursa. Be aware, however, that pain in this area can be referred from a medial intra-articular disorder, e.g. meniscal lesion and is also often tender on palpation in gonarthrosis (OA in the knee). Most often this is an overuse injury, aches after running, fast walks, *etc.* Can be swollen and tender.

*Treatment.* Activity modification, consider local anti-inflammatory gel initially, stretching of tight hamstring muscles and local corticosteroid injection are included in the arsenal. Treatment of osteoarthrosis (OA) when appropriate. Check for possible hyperpronation of the foot (foot orthotics) and weak tibialis posterior muscle (rehabilitation training).

## Meniscal Tear * M23.2

See the chapter "Knee Injuries".

## Anterior Cruciate Ligament Insufficiency M23.5

See section "Anterior Cruciate Ligament Rupture" in the chapter "Knee Injuries".

## Plica Syndrome M67.2

*Diagnosis.* Plica medialis is a commonly occurring structure from the suprapatellar fossa down to the anterio-medial joint recess, but is a rare cause of pain; in those cases the pain is located anteriorly or medially in the knee. If the plica grows bigger, thickened and glides back and forth over the edge of the medial femur condyle, it can produce this pain and also clicking and snapping sounds, *medial plica syndrome*, during activity. On palpation, a tender induration can be felt at the medial patellar edge.

*Treatment.* Is first of all aimed at the patellar problems, see section "Patellalgia (PFPS)" in the chapter "Knee Injuries". If arthroscopy, the plica is resected.

# Knee Swelling

*NB. All swollen knees with effusion should be punctured and aspirated (for diagnose, symptom relief and counteraction of the quadriceps inhibition;* see Fig. 3 of chapter "Knee Injuries", page 68)

## Anterior Cruciate Ligament Tear * S83.5

See the chapter "Knee Injuries".

## Meniscal Tear * S83.2, M23.2

See the chapter "Knee Injuries".

## Osteoarthrosis (OA) with Synovitis * M17.1/3/5 + M65.9G

*Diagnosis.* Hydrops/knee effusion can occur both with and without pain reaction. See the chapter "Knee Pain".

## Arthritis (Crystal Synovitis, RA, Psoriatic, Septic, Postinfectious) *

See the chapter "Knee Pain".

## Fracture *

See the chapter "Knee Injuries".

S.-A. Sölveborn, *Emergency Orthopedics*,
DOI 10.1007/978-3-642-41854-9_14, © Springer-Verlag Berlin Heidelberg 2014

## Status Postpatellar Dislocation S83.0 + M25.4G

*Diagnosis.* Swelling with effusion after dislocation/distorsion trauma. Haemarthrosis is caused by *patellar dislocation* in 15 % of cases (second most common cause after anterior cruciate ligament injury) (see section "Patellar Dislocation" in the chapter "Knee Injuries"). Always take radiographs – can show osteochondral fragments, but pure chondral detachments can occur; these are not visible on plain X-ray.

*Treatment.* Knee puncture with aspiration (see Fig. 3 of chapter "Knee Injuries", page 68) and everything else involved in the treatment of patellar dislocation. Follow-up to check for fragment/s in the joint (crepitus, lockings, pain reaction, recurrent swelling). Physiotherapeutic rehabilitation training.

## Prepatellar Bursitis * M70.4

*Diagnosis.* Most often repetitive impacts or pressure (with friction) from the front to the kneecap, which can become swollen to such an extent that it could be mistaken for increased joint exudate. A thorough manual examination can make the difference apparent. Common complaint that is also called *housemaid's, carpenter's* or *carpet-layer's knee*. A single, acute trauma can also be the cause. Sometimes the bursa can be infected through an excoriation injury or a small foreign body (splinter, grain), the area is then warm and red (can be glaring red-flushed), fever, malaise and sepsis can even occur.

*Treatment.* Puncture (as always with knee swelling) and aspiration when a fluctuation is palpated. *Aseptic bursitis* produces a transparent, straw-coloured yellow fluid, while an infection gives a more muddy or cloudy appearance – in that case, culture and administer antibiotics. A septic bursitis needs follow-up; incision and drainage can be indicated if symptoms persist for more than a day or so (36 h).
In aseptic bursitis, cortisone could be injected locally. Elastic wrapping and then impact-reducing protective knee covering for kneeling positions. In case of repeated recurrencies, surgery with bursectomy can be considered, e.g. if there is fibrosis or synovial thickening with painful nodules.

# Knee Locking

## Mechanical

### Meniscal Tear (Displaced Bucket-Handle Tear) * S83.2

See the chapter "Knee Injuries".

### Loose Body in the Joint * S23.4

See the chapter "Knee Injuries".

## Pain Related

### Synovial Impingement * M65.9G

See the chapter "Knee Pain".

### Pseudomeniscus, Medial Plica M67.2

See section "Plica Syndrome" in the chapter "Knee Pain".

### Osteoarthrosis (OA) Synovitis with Pseudolocking M17.1/M17.3

See sections "Synovial Impingement" and "Osteoarthrosis (OA)" in the chapter "Knee Pain".

S.-A. Sölveborn, *Emergency Orthopedics*,
DOI 10.1007/978-3-642-41854-9_15, © Springer-Verlag Berlin Heidelberg 2014

## Patellalgia (PFPS) * M22.2

See the chapter "Knee Pain".

# Part VI

# Thigh/Groin

# Thigh Injuries

## Femoral (Shaft) Fracture (Diaphyseal) * S72.3

*Diagnosis.* Significant trauma with high-energy violence such as traffic accidents and falls from great heights (e.g. hang gliders), but also caused by more moderate trauma in elderly persons with osteoporosis, e.g. nowadays to an increasing extent prosthesis-close femoral fractures. Observe that there can be a concomitant hip fracture (radiologically examine the joints proximally and distally to the fracture), other fractures are also possible; in the knee joint (also ligamentous ruptures), the patella and the tibia and other multitrauma injuries. There is usually considerable soft tissue injury, especially if the fracture is comminute, where there is a risk of neural and vascular lesions (distal status shall be examined!), and large *haematomas*, 1–2 l, even up to 3 l, can be enclosed in the thigh with the risk of hypovolemic shock. There is also risk of acute compartment syndrome.

*Treatment.* Admission to hospital in an intensive care unit after high-energy trauma, compensation of the blood loss. First gross reduction of greater displacements, careful wrapping. Acute surgery with intramedullary nail and locking screws, especially for multitrauma with several fractures, sometimes temporary stabilization with external fixation (particularly appropriate acute when there are large soft tissue damages). An open fracture requires antibiotic prophylaxis after culture and tetanus prophylaxis.

    *Children:* X-ray the entire femur. *Undisplaced* fractures are supplied with a plaster-of-cast from the pelvis and around the injured leg. *Displaced* fractures in children under the age of 3–4 years and a weight below 15–17 kg are treated with tape traction with both legs straight up, hanging parallel in the Bryan's traction device with the load set so that the buttocks just leave the mattress.

The fracture position in children of 2–10 years should be a 1 cm overlap (bayonet position) with regard to growth stimulation and in good alignment in the both planes; for children >10 years, however, no overlap position is required. If the tape

S.-A. Sölveborn, *Emergency Orthopedics*,
DOI 10.1007/978-3-642-41854-9_16, © Springer-Verlag Berlin Heidelberg 2014

traction fails, femoral traction is applied with a pin through the distal femur (mind the physis!) with 90° of flexion in the hip and knee joints (supported in a bandage) and 3–5 kg of loading. Children of 4–12 years are managed by external fixation or intramedullary nailing (and in some hospitals also by screw and plate osteosynthesis).

Be observant that *child abuse* can be the cause of a femoral fracture in infants.

## Hamstring Muscle Rupture * S76.3

*Diagnosis.* Almost always from sports, in particular sprinters, but also more and more common in football (soccer, on elite level the most frequent injury of all). Occurs in the long muscle–tendon junctions in mm. semitendinosus, semimembranosus and biceps femoris, sometime also in the proximal attachment on the tuber ossis ischii. Severe, stabbing pain in the posterior part of the thigh, the athlete often falls to the ground. A palpable gap in muscular continuity can be palpated. The tissue is vascularly well supplied and can produce significant bleeding with haematoma demarcation and increased pressure in the muscle compartment. Clinical diagnosis, MRT and ultrasound can confirm it.

*Treatment.* High compression bandage with elastic wrapping immediately, followed by regular compression bandage after 20 min. In rare cases surgical refixation of an avulsion injury on the tuber ischii. Circulation exercises should be started already from day 2, progression of the training via instructions from a physiotherapist. Cautious stretching already at an early stage (after 5–7 days) has, in fact, in scientific studies, been shown to have a favourable effect.
Moderate hamstring injuries can heal in 3 weeks, but the healing process is often more extended, and for larger ruptures one has to plan for at least 6–8 weeks, sometimes 8–12 weeks.

## Quadriceps Muscle Rupture S76.1

*Diagnosis.* The quadriceps muscles are the muscles in the body that are most commonly affected by contusion ruptures, chiefly in sports caused by direct trauma from an opponent's knee. A haematoma occurs either intramuscularly, where *compartment syndrome* (see the chapter "Lower Leg Pain") can be a complication, or intermuscularly, when the prognosis is better with shorter healing time. If the knee cannot be flexed beyond 90°, the injury is often intramuscular. This haematoma can be organized and eventually be calcified or ossified, *myositis ossificans*, a troublesome complication. The pulled muscles cause acute pain, often a great amount of swelling (measure with tape!) and deterioration of function.

*Treatment.* Immediate compression bandage, changed to moderate elastic wrapping after 20 min. Stop the activity, elevate the leg. Pay attention to the possibility of compartment syndrome. Start rehabilitation after 2–3 days for more extensive injuries; active motion should be started after 4–5 days. The healing after an intramuscular injury takes more time, often 6–12 weeks, but an intermuscular usually improves within one to a few weeks.

# Thigh and Groin Pain

## Hip Fracture (including Cervical Femoral Stress Fracture) * S72.0/ S72.1/M84.3F

*Diagnosis.* See the chapter "Hip and Pelvis Injuries" for general aspects. Most often caused by a fall in the same plane (low energy fracture) in elderly, osteoporotic patients, but also note the possibility of a malignant aetiology, see section "Pathologic Fracture" below. Be aware of the fact that a hip fracture can manifest itself with pain solely in the knee region, most often radiating anterio-medially! However, it is important to pay attention to the occurrence of *stress fractures in collum femoris*, which have increased in the last decades and represent about 7 % of all stress fractures in long distance runners.

Most often a consequence of a too rapidly increased exercise dose and intensity or a change from soft to hard running surface. Typically the patient comes to see the doctor because of groin pain with weight bearing, which disappears at rest in the beginning; in principle all patients receive the diagnosis "groin tendinitis" at the first visit and fracture is therefore overlooked! Initially only moderate pain in the groin or referred pain to the medial side of the knee. Acute exacerbations are possible. Important to take a thorough history including running distances – react for distances of 110 km per week or more and/or a rapid increase in distances. Seems to be more common in female middle and long distance runners. Cautious "hop test" on the affected leg provokes the pain, as does examination with forced rotation of the hip, especially internal rotation (see Fig. 1, page 98) is revealing. There can be tenderness on palpation over the greater trochanter.

X-ray not positive until 3–4 weeks after the development of the fracture, while isotope scintigraphy shows increased uptake already after 2–3 days, also MRT shows the typical lesion early on. Early detection is important with regard to the risk of complications. Stress fractures can also occur in elderly people, who have started to activate themselves after a long period of inactivity.

**Fig. 1** Examination of the internal rotation of the hip joint (the foot is moved outwards), an important and sensitive test

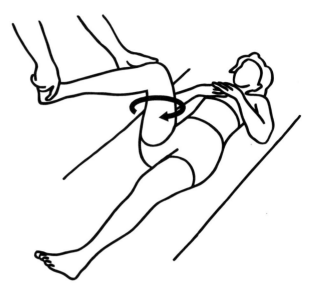

Stress fracture of the *rami ossis pubis* is rarer (usually occurring at the inferior ramus).

*Treatment.* Should, like all cervical hip fractures, be operated on with osteosynthesis without delay, even if undisplaced, due to the risk of dislocation, development of pseudoarthrosis and caput necrosis (AVN).

## Loosening of Hip Prosthesis T84.0, Infection of Hip Arthroplasty T84.5

*Diagnosis.* Tenderness with weight bearing on the leg in question. A pain response, as if you "press at a tender tooth", can be felt as shooting pain from the hip and often down the leg. Can manifest itself at any time during the postoperative stage, absolutely not more common after 10 years, which is a widespread misconception or "myth". X-ray shows a zone formation around the prosthesis and in marked cases "scalloping" with rounded radiolucencies, osteolysis, around it, e.g. at the tip of the stem prosthesis.

*Treatment.* Referral at an orthopaedic clinic to assess the indications for revision of the arthroplasty.

## Meralgia Paraesthetica G57.1

*Diagnosis.* Pain, dysaesthesia (burning sensation, tickling or stabbing formication) or hypoaesthesia over the lateral and anterior part of the thigh, corresponding to the dermatome of the sensoric n. cutaneous femoris lateralis. In the acute phase, the patient can report aching in the groin region. Can occur from different causes in different age groups, e.g. obesity, using a waist belt, trauma and tight fitting clothes like shorts. Entrapment of the nerve when it passes the subcutaneous fascia out from the pelvis. At this point, medially and just distally from the spina iliaca anterior superior (SIAS), the nerve is tender on palpation, which can also reproduce the paraesthesia.

*Treatment.* Eliminate the cause of the pressure, consider local corticosteroid injection and if symptoms persist, with burning dysaesthesia, surgery with fascia release and neurolysis can be indicated.

## Referred Pain from the Lumbar Back, Sciatica * M54.3

*Diagnosis.* The 12, but especially the L1 nerve root, innervates the groin area sensorically and sometimes symptoms from this area can be the only manifestation of a thoracolumbar involvement; n. ilioinguinalis has the nerve supply to the groin. Referred pain from the 4th and 5th lumbar segment may also result in symptoms in the groin, which also can be associated with problems pertaining the entire pelvic ring or a specific site of it.

*Treatment.* See the chapter "Lumbar Back Pain".

## Coxarthrosis (OA of the Hip) Synovitis * M16.1/0 + M65.9F

*Diagnosis.* Pain on weight bearing. In some individuals the pain is distributed gluteally and laterally in the hip/thigh. Restricted range of motion can be a presenting complaint, then aching at rest, nocturnal pain, sudden cutting pain attacks, pointing to synovial impingement, reduced walking distance and limping. The earliest finding on examination is restricted internal rotation of the hip (see Fig. 1, page 98) and then gradually decreased flexion and extension. On X-ray could be seen small osteophytes on the joint surface edges, subchondral sclerosis, cyst formations and narrowing of the joint space. Observe that the correlation between the grade of the X-ray changes and the symptoms of the patient is very weak or nonexistent and that the osteophyte formation is more connected to a pain reaction than the reduction in joint cartilage thickness. It is also worth noting that arthrosis (OA) is not a relentlessly progressive and destructive disease, but could even slow down, so that the symptoms disappear with time; it has often an oscillating course, but can also pass off ("ache out").

*Treatment.* Pain relief, a short course of anti-inflammatory medication for recurrent synovitis. Activity stimulation. Motion training has been proven to be the most consistent method of reducing pain. Stretching for the hip joint early in the course, e.g. in the sitting position of a tailor, standing in a long step with support (and the knee of the posterior leg on a cushion) and hamstring stretch. Crutches for (partial) support in pain-reducing purpose. Referral to a physiotherapist for hip rehabilitation, joint articulation exercises. Referral to an orthopaedic surgeon to discuss the possibility of hip arthroplasty depending on the severity of the symptoms (and not the appearance of the radiographs – you do not operate on X-ray pictures!). Arthroplasty should be considered earlier in the course of the disease than has so far been recognised prevalent. That hip prostheses do not last longer than 10 years is unfortunately a widespread myth – only 3 out of 100 hip arthroplasties have been revised after 10 years due to prosthesis loosening! Hip arthroplasty is apparently the most rewarding of all surgical procedures and raises quality of life and functions several levels.

## Trochanter Major Bursitis/Periostalgia (Fascia Lata Syndrome) * M70.6

*Diagnosis.* Pain in the lateral hip area and tenderness on palpation over the greater trochanter. This corresponds to the bursa trochanterica. Common in patients with hip arthrosis (OA), but can also be analogous to tractus iliotibialis syndrome or runner's knee. The same extended musculotendinous structure is tight, so that the condition should rather be called *fascia lata syndrome*. Leg length inequality and increased anteversion of the collum femoris can be present. The pain can radiate down laterally towards the knee and occur at night. There might also be an inability to lie on the affected side. X-ray can demonstrate calcifications/calcified precipitations over the trochanter at the insertion of gluteus medius.

*Treatment.* A short course of NSAID can be given, but above all there is often a very good response to a local corticosteroid injection administered right on to the bone and painful periostal area on the greater trochanter (a success rate of 90 % is stated). Stretching of the fascia lata/tractus iliotibialis (see Fig. 9 of chapter "Knee Injuries", page 79) can be started on a daily basis some week after the injection.

## Hamstring Attachment Tear (Tuber Ossis Ischii) S76.3

See section "Hamstring Muscle Rupture" in the chapter "Thigh Injuries".

## Rectus Femoris Avulsion (Spina Iliaca Anterior) S32.3, S76.1

*Diagnosis.* Acute intense pain located towards the groin on sudden resistance against quadriceps contraction with flexion of the hip and extension of the knee. Rupture or avulsion of the origin on the spina iliaca antero-inferiorly. The rupture as such usually occurs distally and often at the muscle–tendon junction close to the knee. A palpable defect can be felt straight away, and power of extension in the knee is reduced.

*Treatment.* Unloading initially, same treatment as for *Acute soft tissue injury* (see page 9), including elastic bandage. Then rehabilitation training with a gradual progressive schedule, including stretching to stimulate the healing of the fibres in the proper direction. Total avulsions can be operated on with reinsertion.

## Adductor Longus Insertalgia/Tear * S76.2, M76.0E

*Diagnosis.* The most common soft tissue injury in the groin and pelvic region is rupture of the adductors, chiefly in the proximal part of the adductor longus at the muscle–tendon junction or at the insertion on the pubic bone. Most often intense, sudden pain in the groin or somewhat distally with muscle contraction of the adductors in conjuncture to a strong abduction movement. A partial rupture is the most common; total tears are rare. Repeated heavy loading can also result in an overload injury with later fibrous transformation onto the insertion on the os pubis, *adductor tendinosis*. There is pain when loading, aching and reduced strength. Tenderness on palpation in towards the proximal tendinous area and the attachment to the pubic bone, as well as pain on contraction against resistance. A total rupture can result in a haematoma, and a tumour-like swelling can occur in the muscle area medially below the groin. Plain radiographs are taken to exclude skeletal disorders. On suspicion on malignancy, MRT is performed. Exclude disorders of the hip joint by performing a manual examination with rotational provocation, with special regard to internal rotation (see Fig. 1, page 98).

*Treatment.* Just initially NSAID tablets may be prescribed for 2–3 days. Active rest, unloaded muscular activation and slow progression of the rehabilitation exercises (in which stretching in the tailor position is included), so as to reduce the risk of a chronic pain condition. For tendinosis, a local corticosteroid injection can be administrated successfully, but this often only has a temporary effect and should be combined with rehabilitation training, which often lasts 4–6 months. In rare, therapy resistant cases, surgery with tenotomy can be considered.

## Os Pubis Osteitis, Symphysis Osteitis (TOPS) M86.1E/M86.6E

*Diagnosis.* Previously known for its association to urinary tract infection or *prostatitis.* Newer studies have revealed that an infectious aetiology is very rare. The causes are ruptures and degeneration in the *conjoined tendon* of the abdominal muscles at the attachment to the tuberculum pubis, especially through traction from the rectus abdominis muscles in an overload situation. The end stage can be *TOPS (traumatic osteitis pubis symphysis),* with pain in the groin and in the suprapubic area. Occurs three to five times more often in men than women. X-ray findings very often include the appearance of osteitis; an MRI in the early phase shows bone marrow oedema in the pubic bone. Increased uptake is seen on isotope scanning. Tenderness over the rectus abdominis muscles, most marked over the symphysis, but also over the attachment of the adductor muscles to the os pubis. Pain with contraction of the muscles, relatively often there is also a decreased range of motion in the hip joint due to tight muscles.

*Treatment.* Unloading from pain-provoking activities, NSAID in the earliest stage and local corticosteroid injection can be administered one to two times, stretching of tight hip muscles. If there are signs of infection, a course of antibiotics is prescribed.

## Urinary Tract Infection, Prostatitis N39.9

See section "Os Pubis Osteitis, Symphysis Osteitis" above.

## Inguinal Hernia K40.0

*Diagnosis.* Important differential diagnosis for groin pain. Typically pain when coughing, sneezing or in response to a Valsalva strain with increased abdominal pressure.

Pain radiating to the scrotum, perineum and lumbar back is relatively common. Impact, impulse or bulging on palpation in the hernial gate via the scrotum on cough provocation. In marked cases, an apparent hernial bulge is seen in the groin. Surprisingly common in football (soccer) players (shown in several scientific studies). Can be visualised on abdominal herniography.

*Treatment.* Referral to a general surgeon for consideration of surgical treatment.

## Nerve Compression in the Lower Abdomen and Groin G57.8

*Diagnosis.* In the groin region the nerves can be exposed to pressure injuries or entrapment and become incorporated into scar tissue after trauma or surgery; mostly n. ilioinguinalis, n. genitofemoralis and n. obturatorius are affected. Pain and paraesthesia occur in the areas innervated by the corresponding nerves, especially with muscle activation in regions close to the nerve. Typically increasing pain when sitting with hips in hyperflexion, e.g. at car driving, and then patient often must stop to stretch out the hips. Often diminished sensibility in the corresponding dermatome.

*Treatment.* Modification of the loading, NSAID treatment early. Surgical neurolysis can be indicated in later stages.

## Pathologic Femoral Fracture M90.7F, S72.3 + C79.5/C40.2/D16.2

*Diagnosis.* Often aching and pain on weight bearing during some time before the tumour manifests itself with a fracture, occurs after a comparatively moderate trauma or almost spontaneously. Primary bone tumours are much more uncommon than metastases, which are chiefly derived from breast or prostate cancer (1/3 of each); breast cancer usually gives rise to a lytic metastasis, while prostate cancer metastasis usually causes sclerotic lesions. Myeloma, kidney and lung cancer can also be discovered after a metastatic fracture.

*Treatment.* Fixation with intramedullary nailing and locking screws for the femur, as for the humerus. A proximal femoral metastatic fracture of the hip is operated on with a hip arthroplasty, preferably with a long femoral stem component in order to avoid a new pathologic fracture below. A solitary metastasis from a renal cancer can be scraped (possibly also stabilised with bone cement); a radical excision can cure the patient. For disseminated malignancies the treatment is palliative, pain relief being the most important measure. Referral to a tumour-specialised orthopaedic department for other treatment options, such as radiotherapy.

## Iliacus Haematoma S35.9, T79.2, D68.3, Y44.2

*Diagnosis.* Pain with a sudden onset in the groin and anterior part of the thigh, a large haematoma can put pressure on adjacent nerves such as nn. cutaneous femoris lateralis, ilioinguinalis and genitofemoralis, with impaired sensibility and even quadriceps muscle weakness. Can also occur with a muscle tear that arises with forced hip flexion against resistance or spontaneously in a patient on anticoagulant therapy or with a coagulation disorder. Pain on flexion contraction of the hip and leg raising, also from a sitting position. Tenderness on palpation with pressure, but without rebound tenderness over the lower part of the abdomen, i.e. no signs of peritonitis. The patient sometimes lies with a flexed hip, and a mere attempt to extend the leg provokes strong pain. Ultrasound or CT visualises the haematoma or the tear.

*Treatment.* Nonsurgical therapy, initial unloading and correction of any coagulation disorder.

# Part VII

# Hip/Pelvis

# Hip and Pelvic Injuries

## Contusion * S70.0

*Diagnosis.* Falls on the hip with local tissue injury without fracture, e.g. a haematoma around the greater trochanter. Be careful to perform a thorough hip joint examination, provoke in rotation, especially internal rotation, which is the most sensitive test for joint injury (see Fig. 1 of chapter "Thigh and Groin Pain", page 98). If radiographs are negative despite clinical suspicion of a fracture, a new X-ray is performed within 1–2 days after a period of unloading, or an MRI, which can yield an early diagnosis. Be generous with admission to hospital and controlled mobilisation.

*Treatment.* Initial unloading but mobilisation with stick crutches, gradual increase of weight bearing, repeated manual examination within 1–2 days if slightest suspicion of fracture.

## Cervical, Trochanteric or Subtrochanteric Hip Fracture * S72.0/S72.1/S72.2

*Diagnosis.* Common fracture in the elderly (>60 years), approximately doubled frequency for every decade beyond 50 years. Uncommon before 50 years of age (in those cases high-velocity trauma). The common osteoporosis-related fractures in the elderly occur from falls at the same level. Consider that the trauma sometimes can be very moderate; fractures can occur almost spontaneously. Pain can be experienced from the knee alone, especially when located anterior medially! Sweden has the highest incidence of hip fractures among women in the world (but fractures among men also appear to be rising). At 50 years of age, the risk of suffering a hip fracture at some time in the future is 23 % for women and 11 % for men. Among patients with hip fracture, 60–80 % have had a previous vertebral compression fracture, which thus makes it an important red flag for osteoporotic

S.-A. Sölveborn, *Emergency Orthopedics*,
DOI 10.1007/978-3-642-41854-9_18, © Springer-Verlag Berlin Heidelberg 2014

fractures. A distal radial wrist fracture, which relatively often occurs together with a hip fracture, is also an important predictor of a future hip fracture. The classification is in cervical, trochanteric (with the intermediate form basocervical) and subtrochanteric (down to 5 cm below the trochanter minor) types, where the *cervical* ones in turn are divided into four types: insufficiency, impacted, non-displaced and displaced fractures (the standard classification is by Garden I–IV, where type III and IV are displaced). Avoid widespread, routine terms like "collum" for all kinds of hip fractures on the whole. Patients with displaced fractures tend to be lying with the leg externally rotated and shortened; they cannot raise their leg or put any weight on it; however, in the case of an impacted fracture, the patient can often raise their leg, without help, and at times they even tolerate some weight bearing.

Even fractures of the latter type generally elicit a pain reaction if the hip is rotated internally (see Fig. 1 of chapter "Thigh and Groin Pain", page 98). This examination should therefore be performed in elderly patients with isolated knee pain, even after a minor trauma (sometimes "spontaneously"). Radiographs identify the fracture type, but by apparent status findings, despite a negative X-ray, repeated imaging should be performed within a few days to a week; MRI, CT or bone scan presents quicker fracture verification. Elderly people with hip pain after a fall should be regarded as if they have a hip fracture until the opposite is proven.

*Treatment.* Priority cases! Hip fractures are associated with significant mortality, thus 20 % of patients are dead within 1 year and 32 % within 2 years! The prognosis deteriorates the longer surgery is postponed. Pain should be managed at an early stage. Ensure priority access to X-ray, and operate without delay; consequently there is no need for traction with pin or boot arrangement nowadays. Start antithrombotic therapy, and give antibiotic prophylaxis, the latter not necessary for patients operated with percutaneous osteosynthesis.

All *cervical* fractures should be operated on. For non-displaced fractures (Garden I and II) an osteosynthesis with nails or screws (percutaneously) is performed. The same approach is used for patients under 70 years if they are healthy in all other respects and for bedridden or wheelchair-bound patients, who are incapable of standing on their legs and when an arthroplasty is contraindicated. Primary arthroplasty is performed in patients with RA, evident osteoarthrosis (OA) and pathologic or older fracture (more than 1 week). As for the rest, there is for displaced fractures (Garden III and IV) a somewhat varying treatment programme, where, e.g. (1) a total arthroplasty is performed in patients who are between 70 and 80, if mentally lucid, living in their own home, without Mb Parkinson or any other serious neurological illness or sequelae; (2) a bipolar hemiarthroplasty in patients between 75 and 85 years of age with dementia, need for wheelchair or living in a special housing/nursing residence and possibly (3) a unipolar hemiarthroplasty (even uncemented) for patients older than 85 years. There is a marked tendency to increase the proportion of arthroplasties.

*Trochanteric* fractures are operated with sliding screw and plate fixation; in some hospitals a short intramedullary nail is used, for oligo/poly-fragment fractures (unstable), but also for two-fragment fractures (stable). However, in some instances hard-detected, entirely non-displaced fractures, in fact, could be handled nonsurgically. *Basocervical* fractures are usually treated like the trochanteric ones, but can suffer healing complications like the cervical ones.

    *Subtrochanteric* fractures are reduced by closed or open method and stabilised with a sliding screw + plate fixation or a special intramedullary nail; sometimes complementary cerclage or a specific fixation band is needed.

    The aim of treatment of hip fractures is optimal reduction and stable fixation that allows mobilisation for the first postoperative day, preferably with full weight bearing.

    Patients can later present to an emergency again during the postoperative course due to the relatively high incidence of healing complications; especially cervical fractures are characterised by a 30–40 % risk of caput necrosis or pseudoarthrosis after displaced fractures. These are taken care of with a total or hemiarthroplasty. Increased risk of caput necrosis exists for children or younger people with a cervical fracture, and patients with a large intracapsular haematoma, which leads to a rise in pressure, and for that reason haemarthrosis should be evacuated.

Be aware that hip fractures are associated with *osteoporosis*, and the patients should also be treated for this (see the chapter "Osteoporosis") – "one fracture is enough"!

## Ramus Inferior/Superior Ossis Pubis Fracture * S32.5

*Diagnosis.* Common fracture with osteoporosis as an underlying cause, elderly patients with rather moderate trauma. *Stable pelvic ring fracture* engages the ramus inferior and/or ramus superior of the pubic bone, but there is almost always also an injury in the posterior part of the pelvis, which is not visible on plain X-ray (but can be visualised by bone scan/scintigraphy). Initially sometimes hard to detect on radiographs. Pain of moderate intensity in the groin and difficulty to put weight on the leg of the affected side can resemble a so-called impacted hip fracture (X-ray the hip joints). Tenderness on palpation over the pubic bone in the groin and pain upon compression of the pelvis.

*Treatment.* Pain relief and mobilisation as soon as possible. Treat for osteoporosis (see the chapter "Osteoporosis"), need not be admitted to hospital. However, admission is often needed if the patient lives at home, while those living in a nursing home can return there, upon agreement.

## Unstable/Double Pelvic Ring Fracture S32.5/S33.4 + S32.1/S33.2

*Diagnosis.* High-energy blunt trauma such as traffic accident, falls from significant heights or from a horse, which then causes a crush injury. The entire pelvic ring is broken in several different injuries, the most common being the *"open book fracture"* with a symphysis pubis disruption/separation and widening of both of the SI joints (posterior ligaments intact) after squeezing from the front and a lateral compression fracture caused by squeezing from the side. There is consequently an anterior component with symphysis disruption or fractures of at least the two rami on one side, and a posterior component of a pure sacroiliac injury or a sacrum fracture, or a combination of these on one or both sides.
The patients are often generally affected and haemodynamically unstable with the risk of haemorrhagic shock (a retroperitoneal haematoma with 2.5 l of blood can be hidden in the pelvis); haematuria can also occur, as well as gastrointestinal paralysis, injuries to the rectum and the sciatic nerve. Bimanual pressure on the crista produces pain and instability sway. X-ray and CT compulsory.

*Treatment.* If the trauma is severe, measures according to the ATLS concept. When difficulties getting the patient circulatory stable arise, the pelvis must be stabilised at once with an external fixation frame. In cases of life-threatening bleeding, a pelvis girdle should be affixed and tightened immediately. The case should be handled by a team of specialists in cooperation. Acute angiography should be considered. Internal fixation with plates and screws in cases of larger displaced fractures and unstable injuries.

## Hip Prosthesis Dislocation * S73.0/M24.4F + T84.0, Y88.3

*Diagnosis.* A relatively common complication can occur after a comparatively minor incautious movement, e.g. inward rotation and flexion in the case of a posterior dislocation in a patient operated on with an arthroplasty through a lateral/posterior incision. The risk is highest early on in the postoperative period, but the dislocation can also occur after several years. Sudden pain and inability to bear weight. With recurrent dislocations, pain can be moderate. Displacement of the leg in adduction, inward rotation and flexion, together with shortening with the usual posterior dislocation (see Fig. 1). Outward rotation is seen with anterior dislocations.

*Treatment.* Reduction in analgesia and muscle relaxation at the earliest possible time could very well be performed successfully in the emergency room. The

**Fig. 1** Posterior dislocation of hip prosthesis with the characteristic displacement in adduction, internal rotation, flexion and shortening of the leg

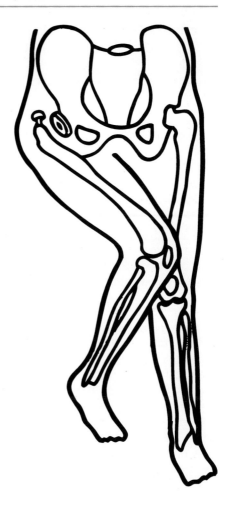

**Fig. 2** Reduction of a
dislocated hip prosthesis:
Note the counteraction
pressure being applied to the
hip and iliac crest anteriorly.
Preferably place your knee
on the stretcher/bed for better
leverage and more power for
the traction and upward
pulling of the leg

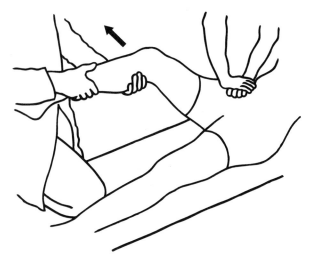

technique is described below under *Hip joint dislocation* (see Fig. 2), but is
generally easier to perform on a prosthesis/arthroplasty dislocation.

On certain occasions you might need to have the patient affixed on the type of
operating room table ("traction table") that is used for managing hip fractures.
Initially after the reduction a certain abduction position, e.g. a "plough" between the
legs and an extension bandage around the knee, is arranged to avoid rotational
provocation to the hip arthroplasty, X-ray confirmation. In case of a first time
dislocation, the patient is admitted to hospital for the same mobilisation as a
newly operated patient. The patient can retain the knee extension bandage for
some time, depending on how stable the joint appears.

## Hip Dislocation S73.0

*Diagnosis.* Caused principally by high-energy trauma, such as traffic accidents
(70–90 %), falls from high levels and high-velocity sports, e.g. downhill skiing.
Most often indirect violence with a heavy impact to the knee, which forces the
femoral head outwards and backwards. With such a *posterior dislocation* (85–90 %
of all), the leg is adducted, internally rotated and in flexion with intense pain even at
rest. Plain radiographs are taken.

*Treatment.* Reduction as soon as possible to reduce the risk of caput necrosis
(increased risk already after a few hours) requires analgesia and muscle relaxation;
thus, general anaesthesia is almost always necessary. In 90° of flexion in the hip and
knee, traction is applied forcefully to the leg upwards anteriorly with some
internal–external rotation movements and counteraction with stabilisation of the

pelvis by pressure from an assistant to the spina iliaca anterior (Allis manoeuvre, see Fig. 2, page 112). On sparse occasions, the reduction has to be performed openly, especially when the sciatic nerve is damaged or if there are avulsed caput fragments. Postreduction films to rule out bone fragments and CT should be performed in order to verify a possible posterior acetabular fracture. Mobilise at once if the acetabulum is intact, but avoid internal rotation and flexion over 90° for 4–6 weeks. Often other significant injuries at the same time, so, e.g. up to 50 % of the patients also have a fracture somewhere else. Consider the possibility of a hip dislocation or a hip fracture being masked by a distal ipsilateral fracture; a *good rule* is therefore to always X-ray the nearest joint, both proximally and distally to a diaphysis fracture.

If there is an *anterior dislocation,* the leg is noticeably externally rotated with a certain amount of flexion and abduction; this can result in a n. femoralis affection (a posterior dislocation can cause sciatic nerve affection, 10–13 %). Reduction with the patient in supine position and traction in longitudinal direction of the leg (and somewhat sideways).

## Acetabular Fracture * S32.4

*Diagnosis. Posterior* fractures can be associated with posterior hip dislocations and occur, like the latter, most often by direct trauma to the flexed knee, as caused by the dashboard in a frontal collision, so-called *dashboard* injury. In the same way, *anterior* fractures, which are rare, can be combined with anterior hip dislocations. If there are so-called *transversal* injuries, both the anterior and posterior columns are affected, which could result in a so-called *central dislocation* of the femoral head into the pelvis, e.g. with direct trauma to the hip. Apart from plain radiographs, CT or MRI, as a rule, is required to map the damages. These patients often have multiple injuries, not least other pelvic fractures with the risk of severe haemorrhage.

*Treatment.* Have in mind the measures described in the chapter "Major Orthopae dic Trauma". Associated hip joint dislocations are reduced at the earliest convenience. *Non-displaced* fractures, particularly in an insignificantly loaded joint area, can be treated with non-weight-bearing, CPM (continuous passive motion) in a motion sledge and antithrombotic prophylaxis. *Displaced* fractures ($\geq$2–3 mm) generally require surgery with open reduction and a stable osteosynthesis with screws and plates; consider the possibility of distal femoral pin traction with 5 kg weight whilst awaiting surgery. Early mobilisation and initially just marking the steps during gait. For some older patients a primary hip arthroplasty can be effective in connection with the fracture treatment, if the acetabulum is not too demolished.

## Pelvic Iliac Fracture, Avulsion Fracture S32.3

*Diagnosis.* Caused by direct lateral trauma, the ala ossis ilii can be fractured, while avulsion fractures from the spina iliaca anterior superior and inferior, and tuber ossis ischii, are often caused by vigorous muscle contraction in sports. Tenderness on palpation over the disrupted muscle insertion and pain on active and passive hip movement. Pain and sometimes slight yielding from pressure on the pelvic wing.

*Treatment.* Pain relief, mobilisation and stick crutches initially.

## Sacrum Fracture S32.1

*Diagnosis.* May either be a *combination injury* in a pelvic ring fracture (see section "Unstable/Double Pelvic Ring Fracture" above) or *isolated*, after fall on the behind. Tenderness over the sacrum on palpation, X-ray often shows a transverse fracture (most evident on the side projection).

*Treatment.* Pain relief, activation and unloading sit-ring.

## Os Coccyx Fracture S32.2

*Diagnosis.* The coccyx is almost always fractured after a fall on the backside, sometimes angle malposition and swelling.

*Treatment.* Unloading sit-ring, hardly ever any indication for surgery.

# Hip Pain in Children

## Coxitis Simplex (Transient Synovitis) * M13.1

*Diagnosis.* The most common cause of hip pain in children under 10 years occurs between the ages of 2 and 12, most frequent between 3 and 6 with a peak around 6 years and two to three times more common in boys than girls. No certain correlation to trauma, infection or allergy. Relatively sudden onset with limping, walking difficulties, unwillingness to bear weight on the affected leg and tenderness in the groin over the hip joint with propagation anterior laterally on the proximal part of the thigh. Movement is limited by joint pain, especially internal rotation (see Fig. 1 of chapter "Thigh and Groin Pain", page 98), but also abduction and extension. Normal blood tests, although a slight increase of white blood cells and ESR/CRP can occur. Unaffected general state of health, no fever. A temperature of more than 37.5 °C or an ESR of more than 20 mm is suggestive of septic arthritis. X-ray is normal (can show a discreet lateral transition of the femoral head with a widened joint space), but ultrasound shows increased intracapsular joint fluid; however, this does not differentiate between septic and aseptic synovitis.

*Treatment.* Relief of weight bearing, follow up with examination after 1 week. Symptoms normally decrease after 1–2 days if the hip is put at ease and are entirely gone within 3–14 days. If the status is very intense, a hip joint puncture and aspiration can be considered in order to reduce the intra-articular pressure. Follow up X-ray after 3 months to rule out Mb Perthes (1–3 %). Recurrence occurs, but is rare. No sequelae.

## Mb Perthes (Legg–Calvé–Perthes) * M91.1

*Diagnosis.* Aseptic, avascular osteonecrosis of the femoral head, frequency 1:1500 children, age distribution as for coxitis simplex, with a peak around

S.-A. Sölveborn, *Emergency Orthopedics*,
DOI 10.1007/978-3-642-41854-9_19, © Springer-Verlag Berlin Heidelberg 2014

6 years, boys dominate (4–6:1), these children are slightly shorter (delayed skeletal maturation). Bilateral in 1/10, increased familiar occurrence. Hip pain (usually insidious onset), limping and restricted hip range of movement, especially internal rotation (see Fig. 1 of chapter "Thigh and Groin Pain", page 98) and abduction (to 20–30°). Verified by X-ray, which however can be normal for the first 3–4 weeks, but then in progressive stages shows necrosis, collapse and remodelling and can develop to a *coxa plana* with a flattened and widened femoral head. MRI can provide early diagnoses by revealing alterations in the epiphysis.

*Treatment.* No specific treatment initially, but increasing the range of motion. Followed by X-ray and MRI after 3, 6 and 12 months. A paediatric orthopaedist sometimes performs a reconstruction to maintain and centre the caput in the acetabulum if "head at risk".

## Slipped Capital Femoral Epiphysis (SCFE) * M93.0

*Diagnosis.* Slippage of the epiphysis in the caput femoris, most common in the posterior and inferior direction, acute (<3 weeks), chronic (>3 weeks) or "acute on chronic" with recent deterioration, occurs in ages 9–16 years, i.e. during adolescence, mean age for girls is 11 years, for boys 13 years. More common in boys (2.5:1) and adipose children, an associated endocrine disorder can be present, bilateral in 30–50 %. Pain in the groin and anterior medially in the thigh can be referred all the way to the knee and also limping. Restricted range of motion, especially internal rotation (see Fig. 1 of chapter "Thigh and Groin Pain", page 98), and gait with externally rotated foot. External rotation in the hip on flexion provocation is pathognomonic. X-ray with Lauenstein projection ("frog-leg lateral position") essential.

*Treatment.* Relief of weight bearing at once and surgery with osteosynthesis in situ with a pin or screw. Also the contralateral hip should be prophylactically affixed in the same session.

## Septic Arthritis (Purulent/Infected Coxitis) * M00.0F/M00.2F

*Diagnosis.* As a rule, affected general state of health, fever (usually over 38.8 °C), feeling of warmth and significant pain in the hip, which is positioned in flexion, abduction and external rotation to bring about relief. The patient does not want to move the leg. Often children younger than 2 years, aetiology haematogenous or dissemination from an adjacent osteomyelitis or inoculation via puncture. Take laboratory tests (also glucose ratio joint/blood, limit 0.5) and a blood culture. Septic arthritis is an orthopaedic emergency.

*Treatment.* Arrange for a fluoroscope- or ultrasound-guided hip puncture; aspirate for culture and microscopy. Start intravenous wide-spectrum antibiotics after obtaining samples for culture, then adjust to the culture result when available. Consider repeat joint punctures with aspiration or surgical drainage. Follow with oral antibiotics for 3 weeks until the ESR is normalised.

## Juvenile Rheumatoid Arthritis M08.0F

*Diagnosis.* Occurs in children younger than 16 years according to the definition. The oligoarticular type affects girls four times more often than boys and appears typically before the age of four, usually first in a single joint, most often, however, in the knee, ankle, finger or wrist, thus seldom in the hip. Notice limited range of motion, warmth and thigh muscle hypotrophy (reduction).

*Treatment.* Anti-inflammatory medication and physiotherapy, referral to a paediatrician, should also be referred to an oculist (possible concomitant uveitis).

# Part VIII

# Back

# Lumbar Back Pain

## Vertebral Compression Fracture (including Osteoporosis) *
## M48.5/M80.0/S32.0

*Diagnosis.* A vertebral fracture of compression type (especially if recurrent) in principle implies an osteoporosis diagnosis. Usually occurs from a fall from the same level or "spontaneously". Women are affected seven times more often than men. It is noticeable that 60 % of the vertebral compressions are asymptomatic, can appear "spontaneously" or just from a minor physical strain, e.g. an attack of coughing. The compression is usually wedge formed due to the flexion force with the posterior components intact leading to a kyphotic angulation, classified as relatively stable, but pay attention to progress of the kyphosis and a reduction of body height. Acute backache, limited walking ability, may even have difficulties standing, but very seldom any neurological abnormalities. Tenderness on palpation over the corresponding spinous process. Note that back pain can also emanate from an abdominal disease such as a duodenal ulcer, pancreatitis, obstipation, urinary tract infection/pyelonephritis or aortic aneurysm.

*Treatment.* Analgesics and application of a spinal corset brace and stick crutches to be able to keep a good upright position and adequate mobilisation. Treatment/prevention of the osteoporosis (see the chapter "Osteoporosis") for all. If there is persisting severe pain, a vertebral plasty, i.e. filling of the compressed vertebral bodies with bone cement via a percutaneous cannula, or a kyphoplasty, where a correction of the malposition with a balloon catheter is first attempted before the cementation, is performed in some spinal hospital centres. If there are any neurological symptoms, there is an indication for surgical intervention.

S.-A. Sölveborn, *Emergency Orthopedics*,
DOI 10.1007/978-3-642-41854-9_20, © Springer-Verlag Berlin Heidelberg 2014

## Pathologic/Malignant Vertebral Fracture * M49.5

*Diagnosis.* Vertebral fractures that can occur spontaneously or from trivial trauma, seldom due to a primary tumour in the spinal column. Metastases are much more common, especially from breast cancer in women (usually a lytic destruction) and prostatic cancer in men (usually sclerotic), which together with renal and lung tumours constitute 80 % of all skeletal metastases. Tumour-related lumbar pain (and the infectious causes of pain) differs from other types of lumbar pain by only partly being relieved by rest. Most of the affected patients suffer a continuous ache, day and night; even increased pain during night-time might be present. X-ray of the spinal column should always be performed in a patient above the age of 50 (in all events above 60 years), who consults a doctor concerning back pain, especially when there is a history of more than 3 weeks, considering the risk of a tumour or the much more frequently occurring osteoporotic vertebral compression. The definite diagnosis is obtained by needle aspiration or biopsy. MRI and bone scan can be included in the analysis.

*Treatment.* It should be aimed towards the primary tumour; if there are disseminated metastases: palliation. Surgery with stabilisation can be indicated just as for other unstable vertebral fractures. A neoplastic change in the tissue can be surgically resected, treated by radiation or given other oncologic therapy. Referral to an orthopaedic–oncologic centre.

## Spinal Tumour C41.2/C79.5/C49.6/D36.1/D21.6

*Diagnosis.* Fortunately enough an unusual cause of back pain, which in turn is the most common presentation of a (spinal) tumour. Characteristically, pain is rather independent of loading and increases with rest, especially marked during night-time, and often progresses slowly during several months, with exacerbation, e.g. from pathologic fractures. Back pain is most often increased when lying. There is usually also radiating pain, numbness and weakness in the lower extremities. Metastases, see section "Pathologic/Malignant Vertebral Fracture" above, are considerably more common than primary tumours in the spinal column or soft tissues. Compression of the medulla or nerve roots should be assessed, and careful neurological level diagnostics should be performed. A complementary MRI or CT is added to plain radiographs. Of the primary intraspinal tumours, 40–80 % are benign (chiefly neurinoma and meningioma).

*Treatment.* Surgical or oncologic methods are possible in many cases; most of these tumours, however, are not sensitive to radiotherapy. If neurological function is lost, it is essential to drain the urinary bladder and to prevent decubital ulcers and bedsores.

## Acute Lumbar Pain, Lumbago/Lumbalgia * M54.5

*Diagnosis.* Comprehensive name for sudden pain in the lumbar back and sacral back region, often radiating to the hip, groin or buttock, but not the leg. Pain aggravated by different movements, difficulties in standing or walking are common; the patient sometimes walks in sideways or forward bending way to relieve a pain scoliosis condition (bends towards the opposite side of where the pain is localised). Is even considered to be the most common disorder in the musculoskeletal system, mostly affects people between the ages of 20 and 55 and 1/3 of all adults every year! Multifactorial causes, normally self-healing (most of the patients symptom-free within a week), but no less than 90 % will suffer a recurrence (half of them within 1 year). The diagnosis is clinical; the degree of radiological changes (incl. CT and MRI) has a weak or no correlation to the severity of back pain! Radiographs should be taken, especially in elderly patients, in order to rule out osteoporotic compression or malignancy, at least for pain lasting more than 3 weeks. Gradually increasing pain over time, expanding pain over several dermatomes, continuous pain independent of position (think of tumour or infection) and unyielding or bilateral sciatica are all red flags.

Usually sudden back pain, low back sprain, lumbago, cough and sneeze pain, as well as pain when changing position. Can have a positive SLR test (straight leg raising), i.e. pain in the back, sometimes with concomitant neck flexion in the supine position (head lift, see Fig. 1), but the test could in fact also be normal by diversion of the attention. As a rule no neurological function loss. Tenderness on lumbar palpation (e.g. spinous processes), paravertebrally and commonly downwards lumbosacrally, increased tone of the paravertebral muscles. Red flags for findings of lumbago not reproduced by movement, high lumbar pain with L1–2 affection and positive Babinski's sign.

*Treatment.* The pain can be relieved when lying with unloading, e.g. with a psoas-relaxing cushion or cube (90° in hip and knee). Initial treatment includes a substantial dose of analgesics (also of anti-inflammatory type), which then is rapidly reduced in order to maintain a good activity level. Lying in bed delays the recovery; instead an ambulatory and active patient is preferable as soon as possible, e.g. by support of stick crutches for a short time and application of a lumbar corset orthosis (intermittently). Stretching in long-step position (iliopsoas stretch) and McKenzie extensions from prone position can have a very good effect. Sitting and rotational movements should be avoided, no heavy lifting (especially not in rotation). Advise against smoking. The patient should return to work even if some symptoms remain as this improves the prognosis and gives fewer recurrences, and longer periods of sick leave are contra-productive, if possible the sick-listing is made partial.

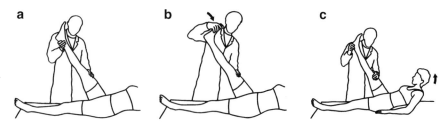

**Fig. 1** Straight-leg-raise, SLR, (the "Lasègue's sign", which is originally really in fact (**a**) knee extension from a flexed position of the hip and knee) may demonstrate a hamstring stiffness (= false positive sign), lumbar back pain and/or pain radiating to the leg (the latter through a tension of the sciatic nerve). The pain may be accentuated through (**b**) dorsal extension of the ankle (= an "advanced Lasègue"), and (**c**) head lift. The angle degree at which the reaction is induced is noted

Pay high attention to the situation of work satisfaction, which is the most important prognostic factor. Referral for physiotherapy if problems persist. Follow up with a clinical examination within 3 weeks.

## Sciatica * M54.3

## Lumbar Radiculopathy * M54.4

*Diagnosis.* Sciatica signifies pain with radiation in one or both legs, most often passing the knee level. If the pain follows the area of distribution for a nerve root, it is called *rhizopathy*, most common from the L5 or S1 nerve roots. Neurological loss, such as sensibility, reflex or motor function decrease to paresis/palsy, can occur. *Lumbar radiculopathy* signifies that both lumbar and radicular pain exist; one of which usually dominates the clinical presentation, could start with back pain, which as time goes, changes to or is combined with sciatica. Multifactorial causes, among them disc herniation (considered most common), facet joint disease, displacement of vertebral fracture, vertebral compression, spondylolysis/spondylolisthesis, tumour and spinal stenosis; new research also points to immunological aetiologies (!). Straight leg raising (SLR; see Fig. 1) produces radicular pain on the affected side (= ipsilaterally, sometimes also crossed, i.e. on the contralateral side); pain usually occurs between 15° and 80°, exacerbated by dorsal extension of the ankle and/or flexion of the neck with head lift. Observe, however, that a source of error in the SLR test is stiffness in the hamstring muscles at the posterior part of the thigh, which can produce a marked pain reaction there. Tenderness on palpation over the corresponding spinous process/processes and interestingly enough on palpation of the nerve in the popliteal fossa, which sometimes elicits a pain reaction felt only in the back!

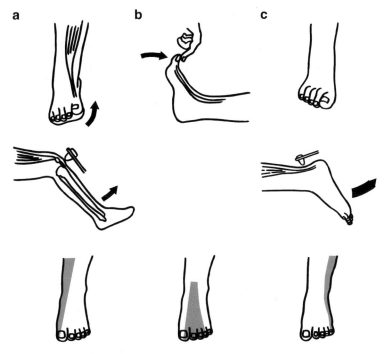

**Fig. 2** Nerve compression syndromes emanating from the lumbar back, neurologic scheme of typical motor findings, reflex and sensory signs (from the *left*): (**a**) The L4-root (tibialis anterior), (**b**) the L5-root (extensor hallucis longus) and (**c**) the S1-root (gastrocnemius–soleus, heel-raising/ tip toeing)

Typically, the root pain from S1 is felt on the posterior side of the calf and heel, from L5 laterally on the lower leg and from L4 on the dorsum of the foot and anterior region of the knee (see Fig. 2). It could happen that the patient consults a doctor only for a peripheral pain, such as over the lower leg or foot.

Pain is exacerbated by sitting, coughing, bearing down, straining at stools or any other Valsalva manoeuvre. In very rare cases *cauda equina syndrome (CES)* with severe, often bilateral sciatica, marked neurological disturbances, urinary retention, saddle anaesthesia and bowel dysfunction; sphincter function should be examined by rectal palpation. It is worth noting that a urinary retention can also be a consequence of inhibited bladder function due to pain. Tenderness to percussion at the affected level, not seldom with sciatic radiation. The sensibility impairment, as a rule, follows the distribution of the affected nerve root dermatome, but not always, sometimes hard to interpret with overlapping. Lameness, gait with flexed body or standing in position to relieve "sciatic scoliosis" (leaning away from the side of pain) is often seen. CT is the primary radiographic method for continued investigation of sciatica; an MRI is indicated if the root symptoms are not suspected to be caused by disc herniation.

*Treatment.* Same as for lumbago when appropriate, see section "Acute Lumbar Pain, Lumbago/Lumbalgia" above. Strong analgesics are given for a day or so, then phased out and followed by a short course of NSAIDs. Encourage physical activity, and inform the patient that the vast majority will recover without surgery.

## Disc Herniation * M51.1K

*Diagnosis.* Same presentation as for section "Lumbar Radiculopathy", see above, most common between the ages of 40 and 50. One should be aware of the fact that a herniated disc can be totally asymptomatic. Even large herniations are discovered en passant on MRIs performed for other reasons, and the patient can be entirely without any history of expected back pain, with or without root symptoms! When the nucleus pulposus prolapses into the nerve root canal, an autoimmune reaction can arise, which is considered to be the reason for the sciatic picture. The typical symptom of lumbar disc herniation is sciatica, where "real" radiculopathic pain usually radiates below the knee level. Disc hernias can occur at all levels in the spinal column, but practically clinically almost only in association with the three lowest lumbar discs (see Fig. 2, page 125).

Restricted range of motion in the back and often pain fixation of the lumbar back with straightened lordosis, but pain scoliosis posture. Symptoms of neurological loss are in fact often missing in many disc herniation patients. The neurological level determination can vary depending on anatomy and anomalies, but also due to compression of several nerve roots. When assessing motor function, attention must be paid to the fact that a pain inhibition effect as such can lead to an apparent weakness and difficulty to activate the muscles. Passive straight-leg-raise test (SLR, Lasègue's test, see Fig. 1, page 124) is considered positive when pain radiation reaches below knee level. Root pain occurring already at 20–30° of hip flexion is indicative of disc herniation, while a pain reaction over 60–70° is of no greater conclusive value. In 1/5 of cases with disc herniation, so-called crossed Lasègue occurs, i.e. sciatic pain on the affected side when lifting the contralateral leg. Ely's test or "reversed Lasègue" with the patient in a prone position, where the affected leg is lifted with one hand around the knee and the other pressing down and fixating the pelvis, produces a pain reaction along the front of the thigh for disc herniation with nerve compression above the L4 level.

*Treatment.* Disc herniation as such is no absolute indication for surgery; instead symptom severity is crucial. It is a widespread misconception, *a myth*, that patients with herniated discs should avoid weight bearing and be recommended bed rest; however, this instead prolongs the recovery time according to all studies on the subject. The most important thing is to be up on the legs ambulatory. This is also true for surgically treated patient groups; the degree of physical activity is the only strong factor associated with the treatment result.

For treatment in other respects, see section "Sciatica", "Lumbar radiculopathy" above. Physiotherapists can try autotraction and, e.g. the McKenzie technique, especially in extension. Cauda equina syndrome (= loss of urinary bladder sensory, overflow incontinence or urinary retention, reduced sphincter tone and saddle anaesthesia) and rapidly occurring fibular/peroneal paresis in sciatica should lead to prompt surgical assessment.

## Facet Joint-Related Pain M54.5

*Diagnosis.* Lumbar pain, which can also produce referred pain in the groin, is more continuous in character and can radiate, but is, without exception, mechanically induced from movement. Extension and sideways bending are painful, local tenderness to pressure over the facet joints can be present, but actually no paresthesias or numbness. X-ray shows hypertrophic osteoarthritis (OA), an MRI can demonstrate synovial cysts also.

*Treatment.* Same as for "Acute Lumbago", see section above. Physiotherapy with manipulative moments can be tried, as well as McKenzie flexion exercises. Local injection of corticosteroids in the facet joints (with radiological guidance) often gives marked short-term relief.

## Lateral Nerve Root Canal Entrapment (including Sciatica) M54.3/M54.4

*Diagnosis.* Back pain, and almost invariably root pain down the leg, which is worsened by extension or walking, relief when sitting down or leaning over a chair or table, or a similar position. SLR ("Lasègue"; see Fig. 1, page 124) may be positive, but is usually negative.
Entrapment of the nerve root in the lateral canal is usually caused by a lateral or degenerated disc and hypertrophy of the facet joints due to osteoarthrosis (OA), which is seen on X-ray.

*Treatment.* As for other lumbago–sciatic pain, see section "Lumbar Radiculopathy" above. Traction and flexion manipulations or mobilisations can be tried. Surgically, laminectomy is usually the preferred treatment.

## Spondyloarthrosis (Spondylosis) M47.0

*Diagnosis.* Comprehensive radiological term for degenerative conditions in the back with reduction of disc height, osteophytes (e.g. anteriorly) and facet joint arthrosis ("osteoarthritis"). The degree of the radiological changes has a weak, or no, relation at all with pain and back problems. This includes CT and MRI findings when examining the normal population. There are even authorities within spinal disorders who claim that the diagnosis spondylosis hardly has any correlation at all with actual morbidity! There is also no simple relation between occupational loading and acute back pain and only a weak association with future back problems.

*Treatment.* Physical activity with a training programme, always including strength and endurance exercises. A 30-min jogging session is stated to be beneficial for disc and cartilage conditioning. Symptomatic therapy in the acute phase. Never use the totally misleading term "worn-out back"!

## Spondylolysis M43.0, M47.8

### Spondylolisthesis (Stable, Unstable) * M43.1, Q76.2

*Diagnosis.* A defect, a lysis, in the vertebral arch (pars interarticularis), that is present in 7 % of the adult population in the western world, can occur in younger persons as a stress fracture in relation to sports, especially from intensive hyperextension exercises, rotation and torsion, as in gymnastics ("gymnast's back"), but also in throwing sports. This can lead to an anteroposterior vertebral translation, "-olisthesis", in younger persons most often at the L5–S1 level, but in those older than 40 years (more common in females), a consequence of degenerative changes in the facet joints and intervertebral disc, most often at the L4–5 level. It is estimated that only 10 % of people with spondylolysis have symptoms. The slip, usually an anterior displacement of the superior vertebra, can increase in children and youths, but almost never in adults. No connection exists between spondylolysis on radiographs and symptoms in the adulthood. The symptoms include low back pain with gluteal and femoral radiation. The condition deteriorates with activity during the day; sciatica can occur. There is also often a feeling of cramp in the erector spinae and the hamstrings. Children can show the Phalen–Dickson syndrome with gait abnormality and hamstring contracture. In elderly persons symptoms similar to spinal stenosis can occur; there might also be back pain when bending, lifting or rotating (from a certain vertebral instability). Hyperlordosis can be present, and with a greater slip, a "shelf" or a (staircase) "step" can be palpated in relation to the spinal processes. Lateral projection on X-ray will display the spondylolisthesis and the grade of the slip. The defect in the vertebral arch will be most evident on CT.

*Treatment.* Analgesics and corset are tried initially; flexion training, abdominal muscle exercises and hamstring stretching are recommended. Repetitive backward bending and pain evoking moments in, e.g. gymnastics should be avoided. If problems are severe and protracted, especially when there is a progressive slip (very rare), surgery with fusion can be performed.

## Discitis * M46.4, M46.3

*Diagnosis.* Occurs as a postoperative infection or haematogenously spread (the latter most common in children). Pain is the dominating symptom, usually severe and with lumbar localisation, but can radiate out to the hips, flanks or genitals. The pain is typically mechanical, i.e. related to motion, and is alleviated by immobilisation. Can, however, have a colic-like course with muscle spasm. The straight-leg-raise test (SLR; see Fig. 1, page 124) often presents a restricted range of motion due to a hamstring cramp; neurological deficits are uncommon. About half of patients have a fever, which seldom runs high, while SR and CRP are, as a rule, significantly elevated. Plain X-ray is normal in the acute phase, but some weeks later bone resorption and irregularities are seen in the vertebral end plate; there is also narrowing of the disc, which typically, in contrast to tumours, is gradually destroyed. Blood cultures are infrequently positive, but fluoroscope-assisted puncture of the site and aspiration yields positive cultures in 50–70 % of cases.

*Treatment.* Intermittent i.v. infusion of antibiotics and gradual mobilisation with the support of a corset brace. If the clinical picture improves and CRP decreases, switch to oral antibiotics, and treat for 6–12 weeks.

## Septic Spondylitis * M46.2

*Diagnosis.* Infection of the vertebrae, generally in the vertebral body itself, but can be hard to distinguish from discitis (see section "Discitis" above). Produces back pain with motion and at rest progresses over 1–2 weeks. Especially affects elderly patients with other signs of infection (e.g. in the skin, urinary tract and airways) and intravenous narcotic drug users (haematogenous spread). Via referred or radicular pain, spondylitis can simulate abdominal or thoracic diseases, particularly when the patient's general condition is decreased. Examination reveals pain restricted range of motion, tenderness over affected vertebrae and muscle spasm. Radiographs do not show changes until 2–6 weeks; MRI is the standard method of diagnosing spinal infections. Blood cultures are positive in perhaps half of the cases, but a reliable diagnosis is reached via X-ray-guided needle aspiration (prior to initiation of antimicrobial therapy).

*Treatment.* Initial treatment with intravenous antibiotics, then continued oral medication, often for several months. If an epidural abscess is formed (can produce neurological deficits), the infection is treated surgically, as is the case for compression of the medulla/spinal cord and large lytic destructions with sequesters.

## Spinal Stenosis * M48.0K, M48.8K

*Diagnosis.* Narrowing of the spinal canal, most often due to degenerative changes in the elderly, presents on average around the age of 65, with disc degeneration and accompanying osteophytes, facet joint osteoarthrosis and thickening of the lig. flavum, which causes the narrowing, but can also be of constitutional origin. The cardinal symptom is limited walking distance with pseudoclaudication, i.e. complaints that resemble vascular claudicatio intermittens, calf fatigue and sometimes neurogenic referred pain.

Typically effort-related pain, with gait difficulties, numbness and relief by flexion of the back (when the spinal canal is widened). Relieved in sitting or stooping, some patients can bicycle without difficulty, despite a marked limited walking distance. Some spontaneously walk forward bended. Can have negligible findings on physical examination and, e.g. most often negative straight-leg-raise test (SLR, see Fig. 1, page 124). Normal reflexes, although some can have impaired patellar reflexes, radiating pain, paresthesia, and morning stiffness. The diagnosis is made by CT or MRI ($<$75 mm$^2$ cross-section area of the dural sack confirms central spinal stenosis). Plain X-ray is first taken to reveal possible signs of a tumour or other lesions, and the degenerative changes are thereby also exposed. The combination of spinal stenosis and coxarthrosis (OA of the hip) is common.

*Treatment.* Analgesics and anti-inflammatory medication in the acute phase, exercise (preferably with spinal flexion) including strength exercises for paraspinal and abdominal muscles and avoidance of confinement to bed (can sleep in a huddled up side position similar to foetal position). Surgery, with decompressive laminectomy, is indicated if conservative treatment fails or if symptoms are severe, especially if the walking distance is less than 200–300 m. Faster assessment if there are signs of cauda equina syndrome.

## Ankylosing Spondylitis (Mb Bechterew, Pelvospondylitis Ossificans) M45.9

*Diagnosis.* This ankylosing, inflammatory disease most often (in 60 % of the cases) presents with stiffness in the lumbosacral back and back pain, both of gradually progressive character. Typically pain at night and morning stiffness that diminishes during the day and with physical activity.

Most often pain over the entire spinal column and the sacroiliac joints. More often men than women (5:1), begins in the age of 15–30 years, almost never after 40. Hereditary, multifactorial condition, where the value of a positive HLA B-27 test (90 % of the Bechterew patients) still does not have any discriminative importance, since 8 % of the normal population are positive. Presentation can also include recurrent eye inflammations (iridocyclitis) and affliction of major joints (hip and shoulder) and finger joints with diffuse swelling, so-called sausage digit, as well as enthesopathies (in and around the tendon insertions). Gradual thoracic kyphosis and loss of lumbar lordosis, which leads to a typical gait pattern. Tenderness on palpation over the spinous processes and both direct and indirect tenderness over the sacroiliac joints. The typical radiographic changes with sclerosis and ossifications (e.g. of the longitudinal ligaments) develop gradually to a bamboo stick appearance, but these do not occur until later stages of disease.

*Treatment.* Pain relief, so that good physical activity can be maintained. Anti-inflammatory medication, also covering the night, can be required periodically. Regular exercise is important, and physiotherapy (including stretching) is necessary, but home training is essential. Surgical treatment can be indicated.

## Sacroiliac-Related Pain M46.1

*Diagnosis.* Irritation conditions in or around one or both sacroiliac joints are clinically awkward to distinguish, but inflammatory (e.g. section "Mb Bechterew", see above, and Mb Reiter) and degenerative changes occur, while pathologic joint motion as a clinically relevant cause has been considered controversial. The clinical picture has been stated to include hip and groin pain, as well as unspecific sciatica, rarely radiating below the knee.
Typically night-time pain, sometimes pain on weight bearing and walking with a limp. Normal neurological tests at examination. It is difficult to palpate the sacroiliac joints, which are located deeply, but a pain reaction can be evoked by pelvic rotational provocation, compression or a hyperadduction manoeuvre in the hip.

*Treatment.* Analgesics and anti-inflammatory medication, but above all referral to physiotherapy, consider a sacroiliac/trochanteric belt.

## Spinal/Low Back Insufficiency (Failed Back Syndrome) M54.9

*Diagnosis.* Fatigue and discomfort in the lumbar back with intermittent pain on repeated or strenuous motion, particularly when loading in end positions, e.g. heavy lifts and rotations. A number of spinal structures can be involved. As a rule no radiating pain to the legs, but this can occur (most often in patients more than 30 years of age). The pain is relieved (or disappears) by change of posture; the patient often changes posture and has difficulties in sitting for longer periods of time. Morning stiffness. Diffuse tenderness in the lumbosacral area, normal reflexes and motor strength. Pain when testing range of motion (see Fig. 3, page 132). Often quite normal straight-leg-raise test (SLR, see Fig. 1, page 124) or discomfort bilaterally. X-ray generally does not contribute to the assessment for treatment efforts.

*Treatment.* Pain relief through analgesics and physical activity. The patient can need a lumbar corset brace, or a body belt, as support in activation, should be used intermittently. Static, monotonous work should be avoided. The patient ought to be

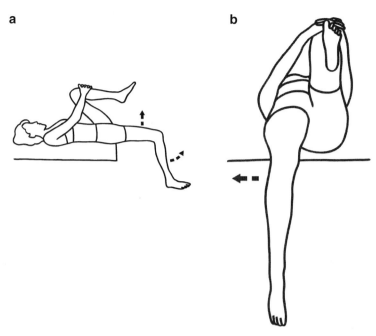

**Fig. 3** Thomas' combined test for assessing the flexibility of (**a**) the hip flexors (at tightness the thigh is lifted upwards), the knee extensors (tightness results in a forward springing of the lower leg) and (**b**) the tensor fascia lata-complex (tightness makes the leg deviate laterally)

referred to a physiotherapist. The ambition should be a return to normal activity within 1–4 weeks.

## Psychogenic Back Pain F45.4 (M54.9)

*Diagnosis.* A strong connection exists between unspecified lumbar back pain and psychosocial settings including workplace dissatisfaction, which has a great importance for the complaints, as well as the ability to cope with pain. In disc herniation surgery it has been noted that neither X-ray nor manual examination findings, but rather a psychological test (MMPI) was crucial for a successful result. Workplace satisfaction has, without a doubt, been shown to be the strongest factor contributing to back pain – influence over one's work situation makes one less pain sensitive. No work is as back unfriendly as unemployment. Swedish back patient studies have shown that a phone call with the message "You are needed on the job" reduced the sick leave by 70 %!

*Treatment.*  Important to take a thorough history and to perform an extensive manual examination of the back, which as such also has a therapeutic effect, while, e.g. X-ray can wait one or a few weeks depending on the clinical picture (risk of stigmatisation with X-ray). Commitment to work and physical activity are the most effective factors in reducing pain. Avoid full sick leave for an extended time, but try instead partial or preferably no sick listing at all. Also, avoid becoming involved in discussions concerning terms of "work injury" and "wear", which is counterproductive.

# Chest and Lumbar Back Injuries

## Vertebral Compression Fracture (Including Osteoporosis) * S32.0/S22.0/M48.5

See the chapter "Lumbar Back Pain".

## Burst Fracture (Stable, Unstable) * S32.0/S22.0

*Diagnosis.* A thoracolumbar burst fracture of the vertebra (see Fig. 1, page 136) is generally *stable*, i.e. the so-called posterior column, with the vertebral arcs, the intervertebral joints and the interspinal ligaments are intact, and the patient is neurologically intact.

As a rule, a high-energetic trauma such as high-level falls and axial trauma. An *unstable* fracture with the posterior column disrupted is characterized on X-ray by a pedicle widening on the anteroposterior projection. Neurologic findings vary, mostly depending on the injury level, where one should note that the spinal cord ends at L2. Exercise great caution when there is a need of turning the patient, who usually is in a substantial amount of pain. Local palpation or percussion tenderness can be found, as well as gaps and haematomas between the spinous processes. When there are signs of injury to the medulla or the nerve roots, ordinary radiographs and CT should be complemented with MRI.

*Treatment.* One or a few days of bed rest can be needed, but be aware of the risk for *paralytic ileus*, and administer parenteral fluid initially. Analgesics, mobilization and muscle training with a corset brace for stable fractures, to the extent that the pain allows. For more severe compressions a three-point corset in hyperlordotic position is used. Unstable fractures should be placed on a plane surface and logrolling used for turns. Indications for surgery with decompression and stabilization increase with progressing neurologic pathology with incomplete paraplegia or nerve root injuries, as well as with osseous fragments that reduce the width of the

S.-A. Sölveborn, *Emergency Orthopedics*,
DOI 10.1007/978-3-642-41854-9_21, © Springer-Verlag Berlin Heidelberg 2014

**Fig. 1** Thoracolumbar burst
fracture

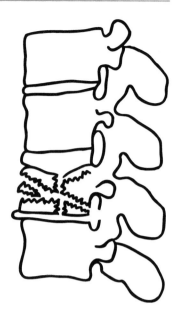

spinal canal, especially if the cross-section area <50 %. As for the rest, see the chapter "Major Orthopaedic Trauma".

---

## Dislocation/Luxation Fracture S32.0 + S33.1, S22.0 + S23.1

*Diagnosis.* High-energetic trauma, e.g. in flexion, with a vertebral fracture at the same time as rotation, often results in extensive skeletal and soft tissue injuries, so that a dislocation occurs. Neurologic consequences vary, generally paraplegia from *translational injuries*, which are caused by shear forces with fracture/dislocation of the facets, resulting in an anteroposterior translation of the vertebral body.

*Treatment.* Unstable fracture with progressive neurologic damage, incomplete or complete neurologic deficit, gives rise to acute assessment of indications for surgical reduction and internal stabilization.

---

## Spondylolisthesis (Traumatic) S12.2, M43.1

See the chapter "Lumbar Back Pain" and section "Hangman's Fracture C2" under the chapter "Neck Injuries'.

## Chance Fracture S22.0/S32.0

*Diagnosis.* Uncommon fracture, which crosses all three spinal column systems, and the vertebra are literally pulled in half with a superior and an inferior part as a result of distraction trauma, when the upper body is hyperflexed over a secured pelvis, e.g. with a seat belt in a car accident. Abdominal injuries occur to a great extent in these traumas.

*Treatment.* Unstable fracture, surgery is usually indicated.

## Costosternal Pain (Tietze Disease)

*Diagnosis.* Anterior chest pain, bilateral or located over one or several costosternal chondral joints. Confusing by hurting both on inspiration (expansion) and on full expiration (compression) or coughing. Tenderness on palpation (with the patient upright to avoid confusing pressure on the dorsal spine in supine position) over the costochondral joint, which can be swollen due to the inflammation. May be mistaken for angina pectoris, make sure that the ECG is normal.

*Treatment.* Avoid chest compression and vigorous shoulder exercise. Local ultra-sound or other anti-inflammatory measures could be tried.

# Part IX

# Neck

# Neck Injuries

---

## Jefferson Fracture, Atlas Fracture (C1 Burst Fracture) S12.0

*Diagnosis.* The atlas is fractured by axial/vertical trauma such as diving injuries. The C1 ring fracture could have components pushed apart outwards, Jefferson fracture (see Fig. 1). Even if the centre for the regulation of cardiopulmonary activity is at this level, and a dislocation involves a danger to life, the atlas fractures are, as a rule, fairly stable and associated with a good prognosis, since damage to the spinal cord is uncommon. Clinical symptoms vary a lot; extension usually produces some pain, but rotation may be relatively pain-free. Lateral and anteroposterior X-ray, including an open-mouth view, CT for further mapping.

*Treatment.* Undisplaced or minimally displaced fractures are supplied with a stiff neck collar for 2–3 months, while dislocated injuries are immobilised in a halo vest (for 8 weeks) and are reduced with such a device if there is a greater displacement. Pay attention to simultaneously occurring head injury! Moreover, see the chapter "Major Orthopaedic Trauma".

---

## Dens Fracture * S12.1

*Diagnosis.* C1 and dens axis (odontoid process) of C2 are a functional unit that together with the skull can be exposed to movement independently of the C2 vertebra. A fracture of the dens can be of three types: I) through the upper portion (rare), II) through the "belly" at the junction of dens with the vertebral body and III) through the body of the atlas at the base of the dens. Tenderness in the suboccipital region can be present; as for the rest, rather mild symptoms, although pain behind the ears and stiffness can be found. Often a feeling of instability at the base of the skull. Radiographs with lateral and anteroposterior open-mouth projections, also CT.

S.-A. Sölveborn, *Emergency Orthopedics*,
DOI 10.1007/978-3-642-41854-9_22, © Springer-Verlag Berlin Heidelberg 2014

**Fig. 1** Jefferson fracture
(atlas)

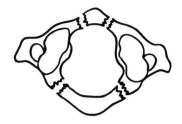

*Treatment.* Type I can be managed by a neck collar (cervical orthosis) for 4–8 weeks; type II fractures can need reduction at a neurosurgical unit and are supplied with a halo vest for 8 weeks, but if remaining displacement of >5 mm, surgical fixation can be indicated, while type III fractures have the best healing capacity and are usually also treated with a halo vest.

## Hangman's Fracture (C2) S12.2

*Diagnosis.* A fracture through the arcs of the C2, usually via hyperflexion trauma, can produce a *traumatic spondylolisthesis* of the C2. Also called hangman's fracture, since it can be caused by hanging. The classic injury is a bilateral fracture passing through the posterior part of the lateral masses. Local pain, stiffness and tenderness over the spinous process of the C2.

*Treatment.* Minimal displacement can be treated with a stiff cervical brace (Philadelphia collar, or similar); for other cases, a halo vest is used for at least 2 months.

## Dislocation/Subluxation of the Lower Cervical Spine S13.1

*Diagnosis.* In the lower cervical spine, dislocations without fracture are relatively common, i.e. dislocations in the intervertebral joints. A unilateral dislocation in a flexion injury generally occurs at the levels of C5–7, but bilateral dislocations are more common.

*Treatment.* If symptoms are mild, the injury can be left without any specific treatment, but if symptoms are severe, a reduction should be performed. A traction device with gradually increased traction should be used for this, followed by a halo vest for 6–8 weeks.

## Fracture of Spinous Process C7 or Th1 S12.2

*Treatment.* Symptomatic, soft neck collar until symptoms resolve.

## Neck Pain After Trauma, including "Whiplash Injury" * S13.4

*Diagnosis.* The term "whiplash" is now considered not a satisfactory term for posttraumatic cervical pain problems (referring both to the injury mechanism and the symptom picture); the term WAD = Whiplash Associated Disorders is also deemed inadequate as any predictive or other clinical value is doubtful. It is characterised by an indirect cervical trauma in flexion and extension direction with an acceleration–deceleration movement where many soft tissues become involved. Several physiological changes occur, both in the peripheral and central nerve system including peripheral and central *sensitisation* and hyperexcitability. Neck pain and stiffness, even without objective findings like restricted range of motion and tenderness at palpation, are most common. A pain reaction often occurs beyond a certain limit in the range of motion, usually 65–80 % of the total ROM. A dull nociceptive aching, often involving a certain burning pain, can start within a day of the injury. There can be a tendency for the pain to radiate, indicating an early neurogenic irritation. Headache is common, as well as pain in the shoulders and the thoracic back. In about 25 % of the cases, there are disturbances of sleep, memory and concentration and signs of stress.

Observe that the prognosis generally is good with 90–95 % recovery, usually within 2–3 weeks, but warning signals for remaining problems are initial high pain intensity, objective examination findings, fear of motion, as well as other psychological reactions and headache and neck pain before the injury. Besides the classic triad of rhizopathia/root pain, reduced sensibility and motility, there might also be long pathway nerve symptoms with spasticity and increased reflexes in the lower extremity with a positive or negative Babinski's test. Other for many people puzzling problems such as paraesthesias, pain from the trigeminal nerve branch in the face, eye muscle symptoms, balance disturbance/vertigo or vegetative symptoms with nausea, vomiting and/or flush have also been explained pathologically and anatomically. Early X-ray, not necessarily immediately if the patient is under 65 years of age and without any pathological findings on physical exam. However, for all patients with cervical problems and musculoskeletal findings, including restricted neck motion and point tenderness, plain radiograph or CT is recommended, the latter if symptoms of root or spinal cord affection exist. Early management should include documentation of pain intensity, stiffness, neurologic findings and, if present, stress, fear and anxiety. This injury complex is the most common from traffic accidents, in fact typically occurring at low velocities.

*Treatment.* The aim is a return to normal activity as soon as possible (by far the majority of patients recover completely), information and patient education. Daily head and shoulder movements, self-guided mobilisation and training. Relaxation exercises and walks. Doubtful if neck collar should be used, even expert groups advise against it, except possibly during the immediate acute phase, to relieve pain and promote normal neck function, as a proprioceptive stimulation.

Analgesics should be limited to the acute setting. Follow-up with provocation X-ray in flexion–extension is recommended, if remaining pain and local symptoms, to rule out instability. If pain persists beyond 1 month, coordinated assessment in primary care or referral to a pain clinic.

# Neck Pain

## Torticollis (Wry Neck) * M43.6

*Diagnosis.* "Locking" from pain in the neck is common, especially in younger adults (and children; there is a congenital form, *torticollis congenita*). The head is typically in a tilted position with lateral flexion to one side and rotation to the other. Attempts to reposition the neck are painful. Occurs "spontaneously" or often after a quick movement, e.g. during sleep; the neck then gradually becomes stiffer with increasing pain. Asymmetric allocation of symptoms and considerably reduced mobility. Acute X-ray is not necessary, but a careful history and physical examination are essential to evaluate other possible causes like trauma, subluxation of the atlas (in children), disc herniation (radiculopathy), spondylitis, discitis, throat infection (palpate adenites on the neck, and inspect the pharynx) or tumour.

*Treatment.* Most often rapid resolution of symptoms, as a rule, within a week. Analgesics and possibly a soft neck collar. Consider injections with local anaesthetics into the contracted muscles as it can give good symptom relief. Cold therapy and stretching. Radiological examination if the pain persists longer than 14 days.

## Cervical Radiculopathy (Disc Herniation in the Neck) * M50.1

*Diagnosis.* Referred neurogenic pain distributed according to the specific nerve roots, with or without numbness, weakness or loss of reflexes. In younger patients (<40 years) usually due to disc herniation and in older patients degenerative changes as disc degeneration and facet joint exophytes with narrowing of the foramina intervertebralis.

Asymptomatic disc herniations are, however, very common (>30 % in the 40 years of age). Otherwise, the symptoms are a combination of signs of pain with radiation to the shoulder/arm, paraesthesias, muscle cramp/fasciculations and neurogenic

S.-A. Sölveborn, *Emergency Orthopedics*,
DOI 10.1007/978-3-642-41854-9_23, © Springer-Verlag Berlin Heidelberg 2014

**Fig. 1** A neurological assessment (distal) of the hand regarding sensory and motor function (from the *left*): (**a**) The radial nerve (the finger extension, C7), (**b**) ulnar nerve (the ab- and adduction of the fingers, C8), and (**c**) median nerve (the opposition of the thumb)

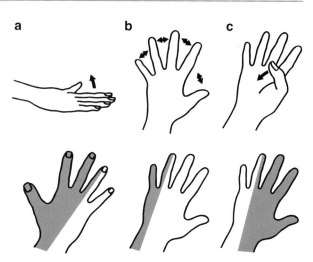

deficits with numbness, reduced sensibility and reflexes, weakness and diminished fine motor function. The C7 root syndrome is most common, followed by C6 root syndrome, but sometimes there is a variety of findings in the level diagnostics from an anatomical point of view. The latter level, C5–6, includes elbow flexion, the brachioradialis reflex and sensory innervation of the lateral lower arm, while C6–7 supplies elbow extension, the triceps reflex and sensory innervation of the 3rd finger (compare Fig. 1).

Neck stiffness in all directions, above all in extension, and sometimes headache. A nocturnal debut is remarkably common. The diagnosis is primarily clinical; X-ray or CT can help (oblique projections) but is rarely necessary. An MRI can give information about soft tissue damage. EMG and neurography are not necessary (are normal the first 7–10 days), but could support the diagnosis.

*Treatment.* Initially as for section "Cervicalgia/Cervico-Brachialgia" (see below) with analgesics, possibly soft neck collar, "active rest" and physiotherapy, however, no manipulation, but traction can be attempted. If neck pain is resistant to therapy, progressive neurological deficits, or signs of myelopathy and long pathway nerve symptoms with extremity or urinary bladder paresis, the patient should be referred to a neurosurgical or an orthopaedic spinal unit. Generally a good prognosis, since >80–90 % recover "spontaneously" without surgery after a few months and most often without any residual symptoms.

## Cervicalgia M54.2, Cervico-Brachialgia M53.1

*Diagnosis.* Neck pain without radiation is classified as cervicalgia, but if there is additional radiation, diffusely distributed in the upper extremity, it is called cervico-brachialgia, in contrast to section "Cervical Radiculopathy" (see above), where the radiation follows a specific nerve root pattern. Often several structures are involved. Monotonous loading, workplace satisfaction and bio-psycho-social circumstances are contributing, as well as personality factors. More common in women than men, increases with age. Dull aching, diffuse pain in the neck (and shoulder), sometimes headache.

Indistinct numbness in arms and hands, not dermatome related. Neck movement difficulties, but passive range of motion, are normal or just slightly reduced. Diffuse tenderness in different neck muscles and typically over pars superior of m. trapezius and the attachment of m. levator scapulae. Clinical examination to exclude nerve root compression and referred pain from other organs. X-ray hardly necessary in the early phase.

*Treatment.* Analgesics and anti-inflammatory medication for a short time (<7 days). Consider use of neck collar in intervals. According to scientific evaluations, a return to normal activity and work can be recommended. Physical training and manual therapy (mobilisation and manipulation; about the latter, however, there are also negative reports) as a part of a treatment programme. Some evidence also exists for cryotherapy and stretching. Consider so-called active sick leave, preferably part time.

## Cervical Spondylosis (including Disc Degeneration) * M47.9A

*Diagnosis.* See also section "Spondyloarthrosis" in the chapter "Lumbar Back Pain". The spondylosis can cause a narrowing (stenosis) of the spinal canal or root canals through osseous exophytes, ligamentous protrusion or disc herniation. This can (but must not) cause neck pain, stiffness and on some occasions, radicular pain. Paraspinal muscles can be contracted and headaches, fatigue and irritability can occur. The cervical range of motion may be limited, and tender points can be found laterally, and over the spinous processes. Radiculopathy imitates disc herniation symptoms and motor neuron signs like clonus or hyperreflexia and Babinski's sign can be positive. X-ray can show findings like osteophytes and disc indurations, and at times, a forward slip or subluxation of a vertebra with the risk of stenosis of the canal.

Degenerative changes are most common at the disc levels C5–6 and C6–7. Of all 60–65-year-old persons, 95 % of the men and 70 % of the women have X-ray-verified disc degeneration!

*Treatment.* Analgesics and cervical pillow or roll can be of use, as well as traction for nerve root pain. If the pain is resistant to therapy, or if there are progressive neurologic findings or symptoms, surgery could be an option.

## Spondylitis M46.2A

See section "Septic Spondylitis" in the chapter "Lumbar Back Pain".

## Discitis M46.3 (M46.4)

See the chapter "Lumbar Back Pain".

## Meningitis G00/G01/G02/G03

*Diagnosis.* Like the infectious conditions spondylitis and discitis, meningitis is most common in children. Fever, malaise and neck stiffness. Meningitis in adults it can occur, e.g. posttraumatically via dural sack injury. Lumbar puncture is performed.

*Treatment.* Antibiotics, should always be admitted to hospital and referral to a specialised clinic where intracranial pressure can be monitored

## Tumour D21.6/D16.6/D36.1/C49.6/C41.2/C79.5

*Diagnosis. Primary* tumours are very rare (e.g. chordoma), but *metastases* much more common, above all from breast or prostate cancer.
Deep, dull and unspecified local pain varies during the day and often worse at night. If there is neurological affection, paraesthesia, numbness, weakness/paresis and long pathway nerve symptoms (lower extremity and trunk) might be present. X-ray, MRI and blood tests (including SR and electrophoresis) if a tumour is suspected.

*Treatment.* Referral to oncologist or orthopaedic tumour/neurosurgical clinic

## Myofascial Pain M54.2

*Diagnosis.* A specific pain condition, *myofascial syndrome*, characterised by muscle tensions or spasms in the neck and shoulder region with well-defined trigger points, radiating pain (also to the arms) and minor sleep disturbances. Most often m. trapezius and the posterior cervical muscles are affected, but also those on the lateral side of the neck, the jaw muscles and the rhomboids might be affected. The pain, which usually appears insidiously and gradually increases, has a certain neurogenic character, like burning or an ulcer soreness. Often other symptoms develop such as nausea, sensation of cold/asymmetric chills, numbness, headache and tinnitus, but also referred pain, limited range of motion, weakness and autonomic phenomena.

*Treatment.* Referral to a physiotherapist. A multi-professional approach is often needed (so-called multimodal rehabilitation, MMR) with treatment on several fronts at the same time, e.g. stretching, blockades, acupressure and intramuscular trigger point stimulation including fine needle technique (dry needling). Special neck pillow/head cushion may be tried in bed. Physical exercise is recommended: "better little and often than much and seldom"! Observe that trapezius muscle tension can be a secondary phenomena to other primary, physical and mental, causes.

## Psychogenic Neck Pain M45.4

*Diagnosis.* See also the chapter "Lumbar Back Pain", as well as the statement in the previous paragraph concerning muscle spasm or tension as a secondary reaction to other conditions of both physical and psychological type. Symptoms like fatigue, difficulties to concentrate, vertigo, tinnitus and nausea can indicate stress-related pain.

*Treatment.* It is not possible to "rest" the pain away; the most important thing is to keep active and as quickly as possible resume normal activity: Movement is pain relieving and tension releasing. The pain could be reduced by analgesics in order to resume activity. Treat the basic cause of neck pain, when appropriate by multi-modal (possibly including cognitive) therapy.

# Shoulder Injuries

*Some important general advice regarding shoulder injuries and disorders: Be (as always) careful when taking the **patient's history** – it is claimed that about 80 % of all shoulder pain diagnoses can be made from the patient history alone. Ordinary **X-ray** images of the shoulder should always be included in the analysis of shoulder complaints. In principle, all shoulder patients should have **training instructions** with home exercises for daily training, especially regarding the **rotator cuff muscles**, with internal and external rotation exercises with rubber band resistance (see Fig. 1), since shoulder pain inhibits the shoulder musculature (26 muscles around the shoulder!) through reflex mechanisms. Caput humeri could then glide upwards and worsen the pain through an impingement mechanism. The important common function of the rotator cuff muscles is to centre the caput to cavitas glenoidale in the joint.*

## Trauma

## Fractures

### Clavicle Fracture * S42.0

*Diagnosis.* Common fracture, also in children and infants. Most often caused by a fall against the shoulder or an outstretched arm, sometimes direct trauma and traffic accidents. The fracture is most frequently localised at the junction between the middle and lateral third of the clavicle, medial to the coracoclavicular ligaments, so that the medial fragment dislocates in a cranial direction, while the intact ligament apparatus keeps the lateral fragment down caudally. X-ray in two projections and preferably also with a 45° inclination from below.

*Treatment.* A mitella or stabilisation (Camp) bandage with support for the elbow gives as satisfactory results as the so-called figure-of-8 strap, which was used previously. Bandage use (also with collar and cuff sling) during 1–3 weeks for

S.-A. Sölveborn, *Emergency Orthopedics*,
DOI 10.1007/978-3-642-41854-9_24, © Springer-Verlag Berlin Heidelberg 2014

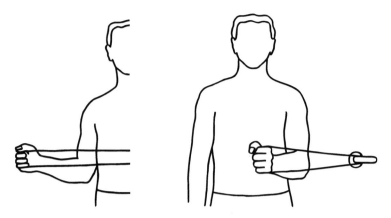

**Fig. 1** Internal and external rotation training against resistance (rubber expander) for the rotator cuff muscles with the elbow close to the side of the body (e.g. by the upper arm pressing a newspaper onto the chest wall) preferably 10–20 repetitions in each direction, repeated in 2–3 sets, twice a day

pain relief. Sometimes extended time with bandage until the patient is symptom-free. Only 7 % of cases do not heal, and these are often fractures with displacement of more than one bone width of the Neer II type (oblique fracture in the acromial part with ligamentous injury) or in the area between the acromial and central parts. In rare cases surgery might be indicated: heavily displaced intermedial fragment, vascular lesion (e.g. high-energy injuries) or nerve affection, open fractures and if there is a significant amount of bulging, like a tent with a peg (in these cases one can, however, wait and see – skin penetration is extremely rare), and if "floating shoulder" with simultaneous scapula fracture. Infants do not usually need any specific therapy. For all patients early motion with pendulating movements from the start is important.

### Tuberculum Majus Fracture S42.2
See the chapter Upper Arm Injuries.

### Collum Chiurgicum Humeri Fracture S42.2
See section "Humeral Fracture" in the chapter "Upper Arm Injuries".

### Scapula Fracture S42.1

*Diagnosis.* Actually an uncommon fracture, occurs with direct trauma against the scapula and is seen in traffic accidents. Local tenderness, swelling and pain with motion. X-ray gives the diagnosis, but sometimes CT is required. An impression collum scapula fracture can resemble a shoulder dislocation. Fractures of the canal at spina scapulae can cause entrapment of n. suprascapularis (see under section "Nerve Lesions" below).

**Fig. 2** Total dislocation of
the acromioclavicular joint
with concomitant ruptured
coracoclavicular ligaments

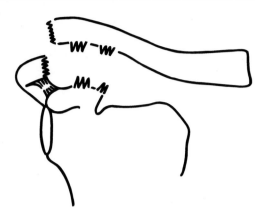

*Treatment.* Nonoperative with pain-relieving immobilisation by a collar and cuff
sling for 1–2 weeks for fractures of the corpus or processus coracoideus, 2–3 weeks
for acromial fractures, followed by rehab training of strength and flexibility via a
physiotherapist.

### Hermodsson Impression Fracture (Hill–Sachs Fracture) S42.2

See "Glenohumeral Dislocation" under section "Dislocations" below.

### Distal Glenoid Fracture (Bankart Injury Grade 4) S42.1

See "Glenohumeral Dislocation" under section "Dislocations" below.

## Dislocations

### Acromioclavicular (AC) Dislocation * S43.1

*Diagnosis.* Most often from fall and a trauma to the shoulder. Common injury in
contact sports. In *complete* dislocation, an obvious prominence (at the "point" of the
shoulder) where the end of the clavicle springs up (see Fig. 2) is seen, whereas in a
*partial* injury and subluxation, the change is less evident. However, pathologic
movability, tenderness and swelling.

*Treatment.* Pain-relieving measures, such as a few days in collar and cuff sling, yet
active pendulous motions from day 1. Hence, early mobilisation. In complete
dislocation, a possible taping down of the clavicle may be tried for pain relief and
reduction. Good prognosis, albeit a cosmetically unsatisfying result for some. No
notable function loss and extremely seldom indication for surgery.

## Sternoclavicular (SC) Dislocation S43.2

*Diagnosis.* Fortunately a rare injury since it can be hard to treat. *Anterior* dislocation with the medial end of the clavicle prominent is most common and may be
caused by a fall on the extended arm. In *posterior* dislocation (in traffic accidents or
contact sports), the medial end of the clavicle may threaten the large blood vessels
behind the sternum.

*Treatment.* Anterior dislocations are generally left untreated since the protrusion
of the clavicle is more or less of cosmetic importance. Reduction by pressure while
having the arm abducted and externally rotated is sometimes performed. A posterior dislocation is reduced (e.g. with a surgical forceps clamp in/around the clavicle) having vascular surgery in readiness. Prognostic risk of remaining instability
and posttraumatic osteoarthrosis (OA).

## Glenohumeral/Humeroscapular Joint Dislocation
## ("Shoulder Dislocation", Anterior or Posterior) * S43.0

*Diagnosis.* Common injury that occurs at all ages, but as far as is known, it is the
only orthopaedic injury for which the prognosis is worse in younger people. Almost
everyone under the age of 16 have recurrences, but hardly anyone over the age of
40! *Anterior* dislocations are highly predominant (95 %) and are usually caused by
a fall on the extended arm or by forced outward rotation of the abducted arm
(hooking situation). On occasions caused by a direct trauma from behind. A
characteristic appearance of the shoulder profile with some proximal angularity
and a dimple just below the acromion. Always assess peripheral neurovascular
status (motor and sensory examination). Damage to the axillary nerve may lead to a
sensory disturbance lateral to the shoulder over the deltoid area and a paralysis of
the deltoid muscle. The humeral head dislocates anteriorly and inferiorly (and could
put pressure on the brachial plexus) of the glenoid cavity, which in turn may cause a
typical impression fracture (pathognomonic sign!) dorsal–proximal to the humeral
head, a so-called Hermodsson (first described in 1934) or Hill–Sachs deformity.
Radiography may also demonstrate a Bankart lesion grade 4 (bony Bankart) with a
detachment of the lower part of the glenoid cavity (a so-called chip fracture), and in
5–13 % of the cases, a fracture of tuberculum majus (especially in elderly, which is
often reduced at the same time as the shoulder reduction). Usually the attachment of
the (inferior) glenohumeral ligaments, including the labrum, is torn off the glenoid
anteriorly – localised along the 3 o'clock to 6 o'clock axis – called a Bankart lesion.
*Posterior* dislocations are much more rare (5 %). They are more often bilateral and
may be caused by seizures (epilepsy) and electric shock accidents and are often – as
much as 60 % – overlooked at the initial examination. Sometimes hard to notice on
X-rays (axial or lateral projections) and may produce an impression fracture
anterior on the humeral head ("reversed Hill–Sachs fracture").

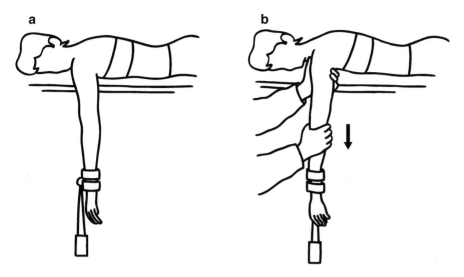

**Fig. 3** Reduction of a glenohumeral joint dislocation according to Stimson with (**a**) the arm hanging down and a weight placed around the wrist; may be (**b**) accentuated through active traction of the arm and preferably a counteractive grip around the axillar region

*Treatment.* Reduction as soon as possible. The muscle defence makes it harder over time. Recurrent dislocations of typical character require no X-ray prior to reduction. For both anterior and posterior dislocations, the Stimson procedure is preferred: initially the patient is placed in prone position on the table having the affected arm hanging over the side with a weight attached to the wrist (see Fig. 3) while relaxing in this position for up to 20–30 min. The success rate of this non-sedated reduction method is at least 30 %. Otherwise in sedation, where strong analgesics and benzodiazepine are administered intravenously and the patient is placed in supine position. Traction is then performed having the arm in slight abduction + flexion downwards alongside the body with either an assistant apply-ing a counteractive force at the axilla using a sling (towel or surgical cloth) – or even the foot (then called the "Hippocratic method"; see Fig. 4) – *or*, as according to Kocher, traction is initially performed with flexed elbow, external rotation and the elbow moved in front of the body, followed by internal rotation of the arm over the chest with the hand pointed up towards the uninjured shoulder. Local anaesthe-sia (e.g. 20 ml of lidocaine 10 mg/ml, "1 %") (even alone) may be administered straight into the joint cavity some centimetre below the acromion. If the reduction manoeuvre is not successful, the reduction is performed under general anaesthesia. Postreduction X-rays are always taken, and the patient is provided with a mitella or collar and cuff sling for pain-relieving reasons (for a few days, up to a week). At several recurrent dislocations, an assessment for surgical shoulder stabilisation must be made. Referral is made for physiotherapeutic strength and coordination training.

**Fig. 4** Reduction of a glenohumeral dislocation with the modified Hippocrates' method: traction of the arm in a distal direction downward and along the body while slightly flexed and abducted (the patient is placed in a supine position) with simultaneous counteraction from an assistant using a sheet or towel wrapped around the axilla

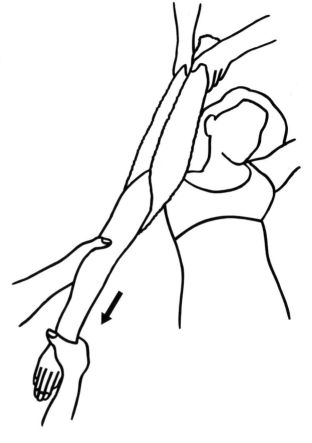

Nerve lesions occur in 5–60 % of the cases (more common in elderly patients), but most of these cases spontaneously resolve albeit in various time (ranging from 3 to 12 months). A rotator cuff tear may occur at the same time, even more so in elderly patients (20 % of those older than 40 years of age). Check the patient's arm abduction ability after the reduction.

## Ruptures

### Biceps Long Head Tendon Rupture (Proximal, Distal) S46.1
See chapter "Upper Arm Injuries".

### Rotator Cuff Tear (specifically the Supraspinatus Tendon) S46.0, M75.1
See section "Overload Injuries" below.

# Nerve Lesions

## The Axillary Nerve S44.3

*Diagnosis.* May be caused by a fracture or shoulder dislocation (in the wide range of 5–60 % of the cases, more often seen in elderly patients) and results in impaired sensibility of the lateral side of the upper arm and shoulder, as well as reduced power in the deltoid muscle, which should be examined specifically. However, the dislocation per se may be so painful that active contraction may be hard, or impossible, to assess.

*Treatment.* Watchful waiting (expectant) initially and physiotherapeutic innervation training. Most nerve injuries spontaneously resolve. Observation for 3–12 months. If reduced nerve functions remain after 4 months, referral for an assessment of surgery with nerve graft.

## The Long Thoracic Nerve S44.8

*Diagnosis.* Despite its reputation, this is considerably more uncommon. The nerve is injured by a trauma or traction (when the head is suddenly shifted by force in the direction away from the shoulder) causing a paralysis of the serratus anterior muscle, which results in the classic *wing scapula*. This may be readily provoked by having the patient pressure hands and arms against a wall in a leaning forward standing position.

*Treatment.* Nonsurgical rehabilitation training since it is almost always spontaneously resolved. At complete tear off, reconstructive surgery may become necessary.

## The Suprascapular Nerve S44.8

*Diagnosis.* Injury caused by a direct trauma (e.g. in volleyball ) and repeated traction moments (as also found in throwers, swimmers and tennis players), as well as at scapula fractures since the nerve passes through the spinoglenoid notch. Produces posterior shoulder pain along with weakness and hypotrophy in the supra- and infraspinatus muscles resulting in reduced strength at elevation and external rotation of the arm. EMG (electromyography) could be helpful, but is not conclusive. An MRI may be done to rule out a ganglion cyst as the cause of pressure.

*Treatment.* Functional training, rehab programme for the rotator cuff. On few occasions a surgical exploration with neurolysis may be necessary.

## Overload Injuries

### Anterior Glenohumeral Instability (TUBS = Traumatic, Unilateral, Bankart Lesion, Surgical Treatment), Recurrent Dislocations * M24.4B

*Diagnosis.* Feeling of shoulder instability and lack of trust in one's shoulder function. Subluxations/dislocations. Difficulties with throwing movements (projectile motions), may experience a clicking sensation and sudden debility in the arm ("dead arm syndrome"). Anamnestic information often includes a fall on the abducted and externally rotated arm. Presents a positive apprehension sign – i.e. discomfort at external rotation at 90° abduction – and a positive relocation test (according to Fowler) when the proximal part of the upper arm is pressed backwards, in this "apprehended" position, so that the head is "relocated" back in its normal joint position against the glenoid cavity, and the patient experiences a sense of relief. Radiography may show signs of a previous dislocation, such as Hermodsson/Hill–Sachs impression, posteriorly located on the humeral head; however, more seldom a Bankart lesion grade 4 with an osseous fragment detached from the distal anterior part of the glenoid cavity (a so-called chip-fracture). Secondary subacromial impingement signs and symptoms may occur, e.g. in a sports situation. A variant is the Thrower's shoulder with a positive apprehension sign, injuries to the glenohumeral ligaments and anterior subluxation/instability.

*Treatment.* Stability training of the muscle corset around the shoulder is prescribed through daily self-training exercises. Referral to a physiotherapist for controls and follow-ups. In addition, proprioceptive training with coordination exercises. If the instability persists, referral to a specialised shoulder clinic for stabilisation surgery.

### Multidirectional Shoulder Instability M24.4B (AMBRII = Atraumatic, Multidirectional, Bilateral, Rehabilitation, Inferior Capsule, Interval Closure)

*Diagnosis.* Pain is often the dominating symptom, recurrent experiences of subluxation, more seldom complete dislocations. A multidirectional shoulder laxity, however, always including a downward manner. No Bankart lesions or rotator cuff ruptures. Presents a positive sulcus sign, i.e. a sulcus, an indentation, is formed laterally between the acromion and the humeral head when the relaxed arm is pulled down. Is often seen in younger people, mainly girls. Congenital with generalised joint laxity (*cf.* the Carter–Wilkinson scale) or acquired, often with several minor injuries. A variant is the *Swimmer's shoulder* with positive impingement signs (secondarily) and aching at rest.

*Treatment.* Physiotherapeutic rehabilitation training (the rotator cuff, the major shoulder muscles and the scapulothoracic muscles) including neuromuscular stimulation exercises for at least 20 weeks as well as avoiding pain provocative activities during the same period of time. A surgical joint capsular tightening through "capsular shift" is more seldom indicated.

## Subacromial Impingement * M75.1
See section "Overuse Injuries" below.

## Rotator Cuff Tear * S46.0

*Diagnosis.* Immediate or relatively acute onset of pain. Generally occurs in people aged 40–45 years or older, even due to moderate strain or in fact sometimes by itself (spontaneously). May be caused by a trauma due to falling, lifting heavy items or monotonous work/training with the arms above shoulder level. May be a result of a subacromial impingement (mechanical). Presents a characteristic inability to, or difficulty, in abducting the arm. When actively lifting the arm in abduction, the patient jerks the arm/shoulder to continue the movement.
Sudden, intense pain in certain positions. Weakness and/or pain is induced at Jobe's sign for the supraspinatus muscle, i.e. when pressure is applied from above to the extended arm in the horizontal plane at 90° of abduction and flexed forward 35°. At acute/total rupture, the "drop arm sign" may often occur, i.e. the arm falls down from 90° of abduction to about 30° with an inability to control the movement. There may still be normal range of motion in the shoulder despite a major rupture, but the reduction in strength is revealed at the examination. Tenderness at palpation over the rotator cuff region. Night rest may be interrupted. Similar symptoms and findings as for subacromial impingement, an MRI or ultrasound may verify the diagnosis. Rupture is overrepresented at a hooked acromion. Plain X-rays may demonstrate a high-positioned humeral head, sometimes almost in direct contact with the inferior aspect of the acromion (a so-called "Milwaukee shoulder").

*Treatment.* Pain relief (anti-inflammatory medication only initially) and referral to physiotherapy for initiation of training including daily self-training exercises (see Fig. 1, page 154). Bandage initially to support the lower arm. If great demands of arm/shoulder function are required, surgery with rotator cuff suture may be considered even at an early stage. However, surprisingly good function may be attained simply by training. At remaining discomfort, arthroscopic surgery with subacromial decompression and revision should be considered.

# Shoulder Pain

## Overuse Injuries

### Subacromial Impingement Syndrome * M75.4

*Diagnosis.* The most common shoulder disorder (44–65 %). May be synonymous to rotator cuff impingement, subacromial bursitis, supraspinatus syndrome, but *not* "supraspinatus tendinitis", i.e. inflammatory, other than in the acute phase (5–20 days, possibly). Anterosuperior shoulder pain, often radiating down laterally in the proximal part of the upper arm. *Note:* aching at rest, often typical nocturnal pain, as well as difficulties in lying on the affected shoulder. Gradually deteriorating to "chronic pain". Experiencing pain when lifting the arm in flexion, abduction and internal rotation. Often an incapacity to put a load on the arm above horizontal shoulder level. Limited range of motion: reduced abduction, often "painful arc" at 70–120° and pain at internal rotation (normal reference value 70° with the arm at 90° abduction). Tenderness at subacromial palpation, especially anterior laterally. Pain upon pressure on the arm in an "empty can position" (see Fig. 1), i.e. in flexion–abduction–internal rotation, as when pouring out the contents of a can. Presenting a positive Hawkins (–Kennedy) sign, i.e. pain is experienced at provocation at 90° abduction with the arm flexed forward (about 30°) and internal rotation (see Fig. 2). A positive impingement test: at least 75 % of the pain is reduced after having administered a subacromial injection of local anaesthetics (not too small a dose – use 10 ml of lidocaine 5 mg/ml and then wait for a significant period of time, say 15–20 min) from the lateral side (see Fig. 3, page 166), for example, and an impingement sign as according to Hawkins is tested. Radiography may demonstrate the type of acromion (flat, rounded or hooked) or a calcified deposit (calcarea, calcific tendinitis), and an MRI may present changes in the supraspinatus complex and rotator cuff tears.

*Secondary impingement* often occurs in other types of shoulder injuries, typically in younger people with instability problems – when the rotator cuff is unable to keep

**Fig. 1** Pain provocation in the "empty can position" used for subacromial impingement: the examiner puts pressure on the patient's arm, which is kept in a slight flexion, abduction and internal rotation

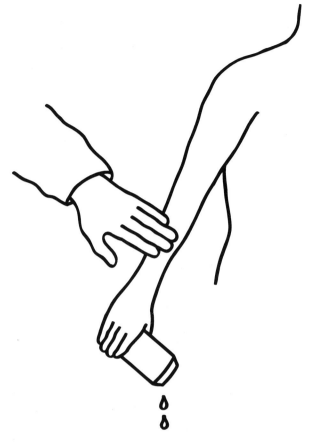

the humeral head centred in its proper joint position during shoulder movements, particularly when abduction is involved.

*Treatment.* Referral to a physiotherapist – 80 % will be rehabilitated through training! A daily self-training programme including endurance of strength exercises for the rotator cuff is absolutely necessary (internal and external rotation exercises with an expander rubber band with the elbow kept close to the side of the body; see Fig. 1 of chapter "Shoulder Injuries", page 154). Anti-inflammatory medication in the initial phase only. A local subacromial injection of corticosteroids could be administered (possibly in combination with the local anaesthetic injection of the impingement test; see Fig. 3). Acupuncture has a short-term effect. Indication for surgery (subacromial decompression, preferably with arthroscopic technique) may arise after 3 months of nonsurgical treatment with no apparent improvement, which also applies at a positive impingement test with local anaesthetics.

**Fig. 2** Hawkins' sign for
subacromial impingement:
pain is induced at internal
rotation of the arm when
abducted and held in a
slightly flexed forward
position

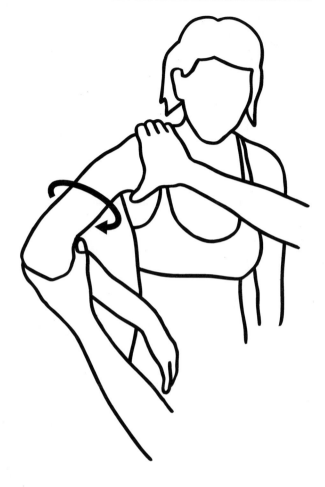

## Biceps Longus Tendalgia M75.2

*Diagnosis.* Not as common as once believed. An overuse tendon condition in a
degenerated or pinched/entrapped tendon in the sulcus between the greater and
lesser tubercle of the humeral head.
Having its insertion on the superior border of the glenoid cavity, it is one of few
tendons that cover two joints. Tenderness at palpation towards the sulcus anterior
proximally onto the humeral head. A positive Yergason sign for the biceps tendon,
as it is provoked in elbow flexion and external rotation/supination with resistance,
similar to that of a corkscrew manoeuvre (as when a cork is pulled out of a wine
bottle!).

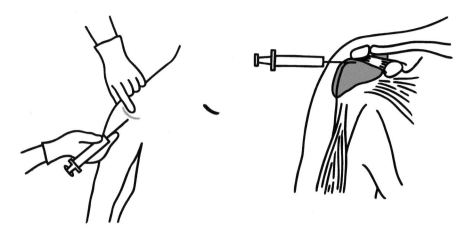

**Fig. 3** Subacromial injection from the lateral side: palpate the lateral edge of the acromion and insert a long ("intramuscular") needle some cm below it having the needlepoint directed obliquely upwards

*Treatment.* Adjusted training with isometric exercises initially, then progression to dynamic exercises gradually increasing the load. Traditionally, local corticosteroid injections have been used, but should be questioned (at least when repeated) considering the risk of the collagen-decomposing effect.

## Other Disorders

### Frozen Shoulder (Atraumatic Adhesive Capsulitis) * M75.0

*Diagnosis.* Occurs in a relatively unusual primary form with seemingly no apparent cause. A characteristic insidious onset of a gradually deteriorated range of motion of the shoulder with an increasing pain when at the extreme positions of the joint during the first stiffening phase, a so-called capsular pattern, where the abduction almost exclusively takes place in the joint between the scapula and the thoracic wall (TS joint). Is followed by a plateau phase of drastic, or almost complete, restriction of the range of motion without any significant pain, however. Then finally, a third phase where the shoulder is "thawed" with an almost painless return of normal range of motion. The entire time lapse is 9 months to 2 years, where each phase lasts approximately 6 months. There may probably be an initial inflammatory process of the synovial joint capsula, which leads to intra-articular adhesions – "adhesive capsulitis".

Then, however, only the characteristic joint contracture remains and most likely without any inflammation, for which reason "periarthritis" is a misleading term. The condition is more common in women of 40–65 years of age, is five times more common in diabetics and may also be associated with hypothyroidism, Mb Parkinson, a recent myocardial infarction as well as cervical nerve compression and mental depression. Radiography is recommended to rule out other explanations. A secondary type may be presented after another injury, and then a worse prognosis is reported.

*Treatment.* The natural course of healing is benign with spontaneous resolvement. Active, aggressive rehabilitation training more often has a negative effect, and also manipulation therapy may be contraindicated. Smooth and soft stretching exercises are recommended through daily self-training programmes (e.g. the Jackins exercises). At nonprogressive results after 3–4 months, an arthroscopic capsular release in combination with mobilisation under general anaesthesia has proved to be successful. Intra-articular injection of corticosteroids may be an option (in combination with the arthroscopy as well).

## Acute Calcific Tendinitis of the Shoulder (Calcarea) * M75.3

*Diagnosis.* Relatively fast developing (onset of up to 4–5 days), excruciating shoulder pain – is sometimes perceived as having occurred spontaneously – resulting in severe aching. X-rays will demonstrate a calcified deposition at the lateral side of the rotator cuff, most often over the greater tubercle (may sometimes be found by coincidence in cases where no pain is involved). Upon palpation, tenderness is always experienced over the actual area, mostly anterior laterally subacromial. From experience, a calcarea in fact tells against a rotator cuff tear.

*Treatment.* Procedure as for subacromial impingement, as well as puncture (see Fig. 4) of the calcific deposit (which has the character of toothpaste), preferably using multipin technique and bursting under local anaesthesia. However, do not expect to aspirate the "toothpaste" through the ordinary needles!
Also, 1 ml corticosteroid may be administered through the needle and a week or so worth of prescribed NSAIDs. At remaining pain, an arthroscopic procedure should be considered.

## Cervical Rhizopathy, Herniated Disc (Referred Pain from the Neck, especially at C5) * M53.1, M50.1

*Diagnosis.* Usually a band-like sensation of pain radiating towards the neck, tenderness over the brachial plexus and the spinous processes as well as experiencing pain at neck movements and head deviation to the opposite side.

*Treatment.* See section "Cervical Radiculopathy" at the chapter "Neck Pain".

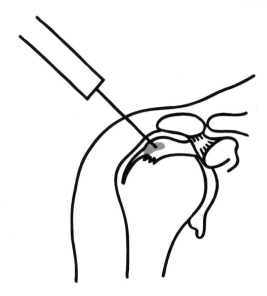

**Fig. 4** Puncture into a calcific "tendinitis" lesion at the typical location of the tuberculum majus and the supraspinatus tendon

## Thoracic Outlet Syndrome (TOS) G54.0

*Diagnosis.* A combination of neurovascular symptoms in the neck, shoulder, arm and hand due to compression of structures such as brachial plexus, subclavian artery and vein at the fairly narrow passage between the first rib and the superior shoulder girdle.

Is often aggravated when the arm is in an overhead position. Seen mostly in women between 20 and 50 years of age, with a female to male ratio of 3.5:1. Varying aetiology, such as the existence of a cervical rib, anomalously long transverse process of the 7th cervical vertebra (both are noticeable on plain radiographs) as well as an anomalous fibromuscular band in the thoracic aperture, but often due to multifactorial causes. This is a clinical diagnosis with sometimes vague and varying symptoms. Usually paraesthesias of the arm, forearm and ulnar side of the hand. On occasions a swelling of the arm and cold sensations. Aching pain in the upper arm, shoulder and neck may occur. Common even in the night. A common provocation manoeuvre is the Roos hands-up test (elevated arm stress test, EAST, see Fig. 5) where both hands are held up at an overhead position with the elbow slightly angled and the shoulders moved backwards while clenching the fists and spreading the fingers alternately.

Normally, this procedure should be possible to maintain for 3 min, whereas patients with TOS report pain and arm fatigue within 30 s. Typically, the patients experience numbness and paraesthesias of the ulnar side of the forearm and in the two

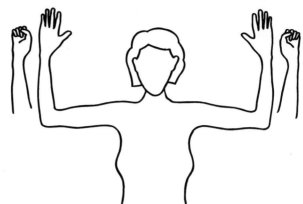

**Fig. 5** The Roos' hands-up test for thoracic outlet syndrome: the patient is asked to open and close his/her hands repetitiously for 3 min

(sometimes three) ulnar fingers. Palpation of the brachial plexus may produce radiating paraesthesias down the arm.

*Treatment.* Most of the patients (50–90 %) are to be treated nonsurgically with a physical therapy programme of muscle strength and postural exercises including shoulder rolls, neck side stretch and neck retraction (the head pulled straight back) for a 3-month period. Lifting and carrying heavy items should be avoided as well as arm activities carried out in overhead positions. The patient should not be lying on the affected side. Surgery would be considered at unyielding rehabilitation (therapy resistance) and presence of any anomaly such as a cervical rib. Vascular impingement, e.g. intermittent swelling and discoloration (cyanosis) of the arm, indicates early and urgent investigation.

# Upper Arm Injuries

## Humeral Fracture (Proximal, Diaphyseal) * S42.2/S42.3

### Tuberculum Majus Fracture

*Diagnosis.* Trauma to the shoulder, either directly or indirectly from a fall on the extended arm. Pain at movement, laterally localised, and swelling. At displacement, the rotator cuff is affected. Sometimes in combination with a humeral fracture of the collum chirurgicum. Radiography determines the diagnosis.

*Treatment.* Displacements up to 5 mm require a collar and cuff sling, and a progressive movement training programme including passive and active exercises for 4–5 weeks is prescribed. A customary X-ray control after 1 week. Greater displacements involve indication for surgery with reduction and osteosynthesis.

### Collum Chirurgicum Fracture

*Diagnosis.* A common osteoporotic fracture (one of four classical), especially common in elderly women. Generally caused by an indirect trauma from a fall on the extended arm in slight abduction. Local swelling and pain and almost completely restricted range of motion. Most (approximately 85 %) of these fractures have a minimal or slight displacement, and some of them engage the humeral head.

*Treatment.* Preventive measures against osteoporosis are of great significance, even life saving if preventing hip fracture, see the chapter "Osteoporosis". Minimally or slightly displaced (<1 cm) fractures require a collar and cuff sling or a more stabilising arm bandage for the first week after which a customary X-ray control is made. Circumduction, pendulating exercises very early on – within 5–7

S.-A. Sölveborn, *Emergency Orthopedics*,
DOI 10.1007/978-3-642-41854-9_26, © Springer-Verlag Berlin Heidelberg 2014

days – and a gradual introduction of more active movements as tolerable but not excruciating with respect to pain.

Referral to a physiotherapist. More displaced and unstable fractures are immobilised having the arm pressed and secured tightly to the trunk by, e.g. a sling-and-swathe bandage. An X-ray control after 1 week. If the fracture is badly displaced, closed reduction under general anaesthesia should be performed. However, at a remaining and unacceptable displacement or instability, surgery with osteosynthesis may be considered.

## Proximal Metaphyseal Humeral Fracture in Children

*Diagnosis.* Usually seen in children between 8 and 14 years of age. Is characterised by a deformation over the shoulder. In older children, usually an epiphyseal fracture of the Salter–Harris II type with a triangular metaphyseal detachment (see Fig. 2 of chapter "Ankle Injuries", page 42).

*Treatment.* A faulty angulated position of 45° is accepted, even as much as a shortening of 1.5 cm, then an arm sling for 2–3 weeks and arrangements made for rehabilitation training. At a greater angle or a translational displacement of more than half a bone width, closed reduction is performed, whereas open or percutaneous surgery is seldom indicated. An X-ray control after 1 week.

## Diaphyseal Humeral Fracture

*Diagnosis.* Generally in adults. Direct violence more often renders transverse fractures, whereas an indirect trauma renders spiral (winding) and oblique (slanting) fractures. Local pain, swelling and a characteristic instability accompanied by a fracture crepitus sound. The middle-third part is generally involved. X-rays determine the diagnosis. Radial nerve impingement may occur (usually at an oblique (slanting) fracture of the distal third, a Holstein fracture), usually due to nerve contusion with a good prognosis. No indication for a surgical exploration before 8–10 weeks post injury.

*Treatment.* Some reduction through slight traction of the arm in sitting. A "hanging cast" with a long plaster-of-cast splint down the forearm, which is supported by a collar and cuff sling and axillary padding.

An X-ray after 1 week, when a switch to a circular two-component plastic orthosis (Sarmiento bandage) often is made, leaving the elbow and shoulder joints free. Start shoulder training early on with pendulating motions initially; more active arm training may be introduced when the collar and cuff sling is removed after 3 weeks. The stabilisation time of the fracture is 6–8 weeks. Sometimes closed reduction needs to be performed and fixation with an intramedullar nail with locking screws, in rare cases osteosynthesis with a plate.

## Referred Pain from Subacromial Impingement M75.4

See the chapter "Shoulder Pain".

## Biceps Tendon Rupture S46.1 (S46.2)

*Diagnosis.* Entirely dominated by proximal biceps long head tendon ruptures (up to 96 % of all biceps ruptures, short head 1 %). Typical appearance of a large bulge on the anterior part of the upper arm due to the retracted muscle belly, most evident and accentuated at attempts of tightening the muscles (Ludington's sign). Sudden, sharp pain in the upper arm, often accompanied by an audible snap. A palpable defect in the upper arm and ecchymosis at mid and lower upper arm level. Generally seen in people over the age of 40, but sometimes also in younger adults. In the latter case, usually due to lifting heavy items. In the elderly, it may occur at moderate loading strain due to degenerative processes in and around the tendon in the bicipital groove (the humeral head sulcus) and may then be associated with subacromial impingement and rotator cuff tears.

*Treatment.* A nonsurgical regimen including range of motion and strengthening training programme as long as pain is tolerable. After the therapy period, a restriction in function is seldom seen, not even in professions and occupations that involve loading tasks.

# Part XI

# Elbow

# Elbow Injuries

*Some important general advice regarding elbow injuries: Avoid a long duration of elbow immobilisation, a maximum of 3 weeks for adults. Children could go 5–6 weeks until restriction of range of motion persists. Avoid forceful, aggressive physiotherapeutic manipulation, especially bouncing, dynamic stretching, which may only render a worse result in regards to the range of motion (e.g. creating myositis ossificans). In elbow injuries, there is a risk of damaging the blood vessels and nerves – always perform a peripheral neurovascular examination (distal status)!*

## Trauma

### Supracondylar Humerus (Elbow) Fracture * S42.4

*Diagnosis.* A distal humerus fracture is the most common elbow fracture in children (50–60 %) with a peak at the age of 5–8 years (mostly boys). Is very rarely seen in adults. Occurs from fall on the extended arm, a hyperextension trauma (95 %) with the shaft fragment anterior to the elbow joint (see Fig. 1), or in rare cases, after a fall onto the flexed elbow and the shaft fragment in a posterior position. A very important fracture due to the risk of damaging the brachial artery (in 5–12 %) or the median (mostly), the radial or the ulnar nerves (in 5–19 %), particularly in displaced extension injuries. Make a peripheral neurovascular examination (distal status) and check pulse, coloration, temperature, sensibility and active motility (in the fingers)! There is a quick swelling of the elbow (typical antecubital ecchymosis after a few hours), pain and instability.
Radiographs should be taken promptly. Pain at passive extension of the fingers may indicate compartment syndrome, although very rare (<1 %).

*Treatment.* The elbow is stabilised immediately with a splint at 20–30° of flexion before X-ray. Closed reduction under general anaesthesia is the first priority in

**Fig. 1** Supracondylar
humeral fracture, which may
damage the brachial artery as
well as the median, radial or
ulnar nerves

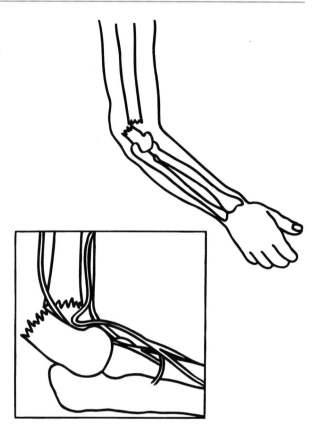

displaced fractures (see Fig. 2). However, fractures with a displacement <20° may
be provided with a dorsal plaster-of-cast splint only – for 3–4 weeks – having the
elbow at 90° of flexion. Never use circular plaster. A collar and cuff sling is
provided for arm support. At difficulties in having the fracture in a stable position,
the fracture has to be fixated with crossed pins through closed or open reduction.
The pins are pinched off outside the skin. Palpate the radial pulse throughout the
reduction manoeuvres!

Avoid repeated reduction attempts. In-hospital care with regular checkups of the
peripheral neurovascular status (distal status). An X-ray control after 4 days and a
fixation time of 3–4 weeks, then another X-ray control upon removal of the plaster-
of-cast. If healed properly at this time, the fracture pins are extracted as well.
Preferably a mobilisation control 3–4 weeks post removal of the plaster-of-cast.

At impending ischaemia, the bandages are cut and the elbow straightened since
the most common cause of ischaemia is due to a plaster-of-cast in considerable
flexion. If the expected effect is not presented, indication for a surgical exploration or

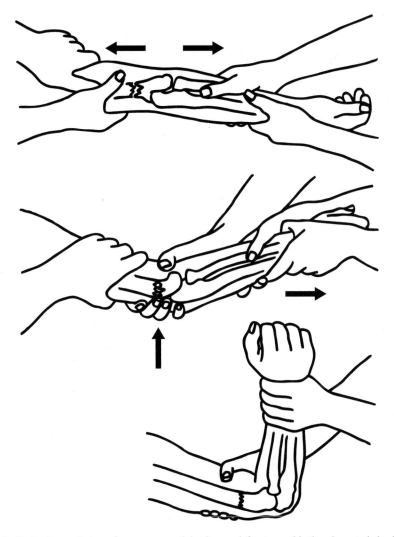

**Fig. 2** Reduction technique for a supracondylar humeral fracture with the characteristic dorsal displacement of the distal fragment: the length is restored through traction and applied counteraction (*upper*); subsequently a reduction is performed by applying direct pressure to the distal fragment (*middle*), and finally the reduced position is maintained/preserved through flexion of the elbow with the forearm in pronation (*lower*)

the risk of Volkmann's ischemic contracture with muscle necrosis and shrinking is immediate. Also be sure to observe if there is a rotational misalignment (generally the distal fracture component is rotated inward). However, this may be difficult to see on plain radiographs, thus CT may be required.

## Condylar Humerus Fracture S42.4

*Diagnosis.* A rare fracture, which mostly occurs in people of fairly old age, is often intra-articular and may be either trans- or intercondylar of T- or Y-shape. Generally caused by a direct trauma, rendering a displaced, unstable type of fracture. Motion pain, swelling and instability. Perform an X-ray and be generous with CT for mapping.

*Treatment.* As a rule, open reduction and osteosynthesis are performed since the fractures generally are displaced and unstable, also because a stable osteosynthesis does not require immobilisation. A general principle is that the elbow of an adult is never to be immobilised for more than 3 weeks due to the risk of stiffness and extension defect! A minimally displaced and stable fracture may be provided with a removable splint, and supination and pronation movements may be initiated with caution already 3 days post injury. Active flexion–extension to a certain degree may be introduced after 2 weeks.

At highly comminuted fractures in old people with osteopenia, osteosynthesis may be impracticable and a fixation for some week must be established instead, where-upon an active mobilisation is started depending on how much pain is induced. Possibly, there may be indication for an articulated external fixation or olecranon traction.

## Fractures of the Capitulum of the Humerus (Capitellum Humeri Fracture) S42.4

*Diagnosis.* Fall on the extended arm, only seen in adults. The capitulum dislocates forwardly and proximally, often with a rotation up to 90°. Occurs also in combination with a radial head fracture. Swelling with mobility limitation that produces pain.

*Treatment.* Closed reduction may be attempted through traction in elbow extension and pressure against the fracture fragment. However, open reduction and osteosynthesis are generally required. At stable osteosynthesis, do *not* immobilise, otherwise a dorsal plaster-of-cast splint should be provided for 3 weeks with the elbow flexed at 90°. At a comparatively stable fracture position, a removable splint and physiotherapist-guided motion training with caution are allowed. Customary X-ray control after 1 week.

## Epicondyle Fractures S42.4

### Radial Humerus Condyle Fractures

*Diagnosis.* Fall on the extended arm, which results in an oblique fracture (chisel fracture) of intra-articular epiphysiolysis-type Salter–Harris IV (see Fig. 2 of chapter "Ankle Injuries", page 42), and is thus occurring only in children. The fragment, including the radial epicondyle, capitulum radii, a part of the trochlea and a part of the metaphysis, may rotate 90° in the sagittal as well as the frontal plane and is often substantially displaced. Undisplaced fractures of these localities may, however, be potentially unstable (due to the muscle tractions). Swelling and tenderness over the radial elbow area. X-rays may be difficult to assess due to the incomplete ossification of these small children (compare with the uninjured side).

*Treatment.* Undisplaced fractures are supplied with a plaster splint at 90° for 3 weeks and X-ray (plaster removed) after 1 and 2 weeks, respectively. At displacement of >2 mm, open reduction and osteosynthesis upon which a plaster splint is provided for 3 weeks.

### Ulnar Humerus Epicondyle Fractures

*Diagnosis.* An apophyseal avulsion (distraction) fracture (not the epiphysis). In half of the cases in combination with an elbow dislocation, otherwise caused by an abduction trauma. A considerable fracture displacement may be present. Swelling and tenderness at palpation, which also may identify a surprisingly large defect from the epicondyle avulsion in the ulnar elbow area. Radiography should include a supplementary X-ray of the healthy side for comparison.

*Treatment.* An undisplaced fracture is put in plaster for 10–14 days. At reduction of an elbow dislocation, the epicondyle is often settled in its right position simultaneously. At an epicondyle displacement of >5 mm, and especially if it intrudes into the joint, an open reduction and an osteosynthesis are performed and a postoperative dorsal plaster splint is provided for 10–14 days. Generally, it will take as long as 2–3 months until the range of motion of the elbow has been normalised.

## Elbow Dislocation * S53.1

*Diagnosis.* In children, this is the most common joint to dislocate. In adults, it is surpassed in frequency only by shoulder and finger dislocations. Of all the elbow dislocations, 10–20 % also involves fractures, e.g. condyle avulsion fractures (in 12 % of the cases), coronoid process fractures (in 10 %) and radial head fractures (in 5–10 %). The injury mechanism is usually triggered by a fall on the hyperextended arm. Neurovascular injuries may occur (more common to the ulnar nerve) – thus,

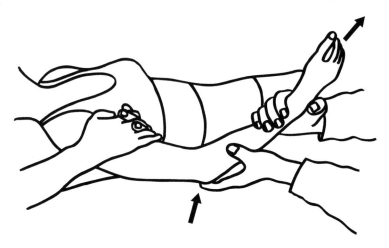

**Fig. 3** Closed reduction of an elbow dislocation: traction while the elbow is (semi)flexed and the forearm in supination. A manual pressure could be applied forwardly to the distal olecranon to facilitate

always perform a peripheral neurovascular examination (distal status)! Generally the olecranon dislocates posteriorly and the elbow presents a characteristic deformation, which, however, may look similar to that of a supracondylar humerus fracture with the olecranon process protruding posteriorly. Mobility limitation with severe pain and tenderness at palpation, which should especially be noted over the ulnar area, e.g. in children often an ulnar epicondyle detachment/avulsion. Radiography both prior to and postreduction.

*Treatment.* Closed reduction with semiflexed elbow (see Fig. 3) under general anaesthesia (always in children) to be carried out promptly. In adults, a combination of intravenous analgesics and benzodiazepines may also be used. A posterior, long splint with the elbow flexed at 90–100° and the hand in slight pronation for 1 week. An X-ray control to be performed immediately (be sure to observe satisfactory joint congruence) and after 3–4 days as well. Dislocation in combination with a displaced radial head fracture or an ulnar epicondyle displacement of >5 mm may require surgery (however without an extirpation of the radial head). When the coronoid process is fractured (mostly in adults), a prolonged plaster immobilisation of 2–3 weeks may be recommended. However, if the reduction is hard to maintain, an osteosynthesis may be necessary as well.

As much as up to 50 % of the dislocations may have remaining problems, e.g. with limited range of motion, pain, weakness and instability.

## Subluxation of the Radial Head (Pulled Elbow/Nursemaid's Elbow) * S53.0

*Diagnosis.* Subluxation of the radial head partly out of the annular ligament, caused when the child's forearm is jerked while pronated and/or by traction (pulling) of the extended elbow. The most common elbow injury in children of age 4 or younger, most frequently occurring in the ages of 1–3 years. The child typically presents a stiff elbow, which is somewhat flexed and the forearm mid-pronated, hanging along the body side, and avoids using the hand. The subluxation itself is not visible at radiography, but X-rays may be taken so that other injuries can be ruled out.

*Treatment.* Reduction through quick manipulation, without anaesthesia, having the elbow flexed at 90° and pressure is applied to the radial head while a distinct supination (and then pronation) movement is performed. Often a snap is felt (see Fig. 4) or even heard, and the child may experience pain momentarily. The child will, however, begin to use the arm normally in only a few minutes after reduction. Immobilisation is not necessary, but the parents are to be informed of the injury cause and that recurrences may occur. If the reduction, contrary to expectation, is not successful, an arm sling may be used for a few days upon which reduction is achieved spontaneously.

## Olecranon Fracture * M52.0

*Diagnosis.* Occurs at fall and direct blow to the elbow or due to a fall on the extended hand with the elbow in flexion. May be associated with a radial head fracture or an elbow dislocation, also seen in children with a collum radii fracture. Predominantly, a transverse or slightly oblique (slanting) fracture lines a few centimetres distal to the olecranon tip. A non-displaced fracture has only moderate swelling, but otherwise often swollen quite prominently due to the fracture hematoma. Pain when moving as well as mobility limitation. At palpation the defect is often evident and a deformity is seen. The extension ability is reduced or absent. Check nerve functions, especially the ulnar nerve. X-ray the entire forearm.

*Treatment.* The more uncommon non-displaced type (where the triceps tendon is intact) is provided with a posterior plaster splint at 45° of flexion for 2–3 weeks. The rest is operated on, generally with tension band (Weber) wiring, Zuggurtung ("traction girdle" in German) technique, i.e. with two parallel pins and cerclage in an 8-shaped formation (through a small drill canal in the distal fragment). In general, this type of fixation becomes stable and postoperative immobilisation will not be necessary. Active motion training from early on. A customary X-ray control after 1 week.

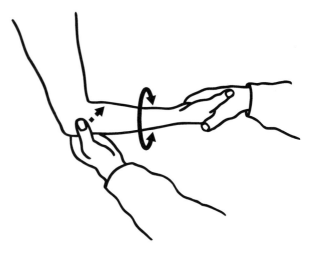

**Fig. 4** Reduction of a subluxation of the radial head (pulled/nursemaid's elbow): at 90° of elbow flexion while applying pressure to the radial head, a distinct supination (and pronation) manoeuvre is carried out

## Radial Head Fracture (Caput Radii Fracture) * S52.1

*Diagnosis.* A fracture of the radial head generally results from a fall on the outstretched hand while the forearm is in pronation, almost only seen in adults. Tenderness and swelling over the radial elbow area and pain at movements, which are limited. May be a fracture of chisel-cut avulsion or intersectional axial type, but could also be a compression fracture with incongruence of the joint surface. Sometimes a combination injury with an elbow dislocation or a fracture of the capitulum of the humerus, for example.

*Treatment.* Note that a large intra-articular hematoma is usually presented and should be aspirated upon which the pain is radically diminished and the range of motion improved (see Fig. 5 and the chapter "Basic Injection Techniques"). Non-displaced or slightly displaced fractures (up to 2 mm articular surface hitch) are most common and should be joint punctured accordingly, elastically swathed and finally provided with a collar and cuff sling for 3–4 days. Active motion training exercises already from the second day post injury. Displaced fractures of chisel-cut avulsion type involving more than 1/3 of the articular surface as well as comminuted fractures are reduced openly and fixed with osteosynthesis. For highly comminuted fractures that are not accessible, or suitable for osteosynthesis, extirpation of the radial head may be an adequate procedure. This may also be the case of nonsurgically treated fractures where the discomfort is considerably prolonged. If an adequate range of motion is achieved within 5 days post injury, the extirpation of the radial head is to be avoided.

**Fig. 5** Puncture for
aspiration of the elbow joint
via the "soft spot" = the
triangular area just distal to
the olecranon tip in the radial
direction where a fluctuation
is palpated due to the effusion
in the joint

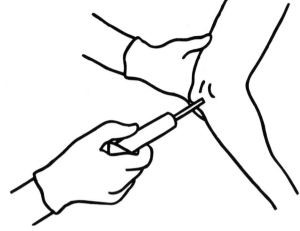

## Collum Radii Fracture * S52.1

*Diagnosis.* Most often seen in children, caused by an abduction trauma on the extended elbow (in supination), often physiolysis. A wide variation in the degrees of displacement may be presented. When assessing X-rays, one should also look for other associated fractures. Painful range of motion limitation, swelling and tenderness.

*Treatment.* Angulation in older children is accepted up to 15°, as much as 30° for children under 10 years of age. At a greater angulation, a closed reduction under general anaesthesia is performed with extension, supination and varus position of the elbow along with locally applied pressure over the radial head inward and upwards, which will often render a stable fracture situation. The elbow is fixed with a dorsal plaster splint at 90° of flexion for 3 weeks. If a satisfactory position is not reached, an open reduction is performed. However, extirpation of the radial head must never be done in children (due to the risk of disturbing the growth)!

In *adults* having collum radii fractures with less than 30° of angulation and no ad latus dislocation, aspiration of the hematoma from the joint is carried out. An elastic bandage and a collar and cuff sling are then provided for 2 weeks, and active motion training is to be performed at an early stage.

## Overload Injuries

### Distal Biceps Tendon Rupture S46.8

*Diagnosis.* Although very rare, this is the most common tendon rupture of the elbow region, even if they account for only 3–10 % of all the biceps tendon ruptures.

Almost exclusively seen in men at the average age of 40–50 years. The dominant arm is affected in approximately 80 % of the cases. Nearly all distal biceps tendon ruptures are avulsions of the radial tuberosity, and partial ruptures are rare. Occurs in an isolated overload situation, often due to lifting weights of 40 kg, or more, with the elbow flexed at 90°, or in a similar eccentric loading situation when a sudden passive extension occurs, such as that of a catching a falling object. Generally seen in people of manual labour/heavy workloads, weightlifters, bodybuilders or gymnasts. The risk of rupture (also a partial type) is increased by the use of anabolic steroids. Typically, a snap or crack with a sharp bursting pain is felt in the cubital fossa, but the pain often subsides within a few hours, leaving a dull aching pain that may persist for several weeks. Flexion and supination are weakened while also being painful. Local tenderness in the cubital fossa where a bleeding discoloration appears within a few days. A deformity is seen due to a transposition of the belly of biceps muscle proximally, and a palpable defect is evident at attempts of muscle contraction. The range of motion is not significantly affected, and a normal radiography is usually demonstrated. At some occasions, an avulsion flake may be observed.

*Treatment.* Excellent results are reported at surgery that is done at an early stage with suture and refixation of the tendon to the radius in active people. However, nonsurgical treatments may also render a satisfactory result, even if there may be a remaining reduction of the supination strength, as well as a poorer flexion power.

## Triceps Tendon Rupture S46.3

*Diagnosis.* An exceptionally rare tendon rupture, it is actually better called triceps avulsion (may be the most unusual tendon rupture of all in man). It has the same occurrence frequency for the right and left elbow, and the gender distribution is more even (a men/women ratio 3:2) than biceps tendon tears. Occurs typically after falling on the outstretched arm with a simultaneous sudden and forceful flexion load of eccentric type to the extended elbow. There is almost always a tear in the tendo-osseous area with a detached bone fragment, and 80 % of the radiography proves to be affirmative. May be associated with a radial head fracture after a fall (has been described as a new syndrome). For weightlifters and bodybuilders, a possible correlation with the use of anabolic steroids or local cortisone injections has been observed. Average age at injury is 33 years (range 7–70). Sudden posterior elbow pain followed by swelling and weakness at elbow extension (the triceps muscle is the only elbow extensor). The presence of a palpable gap proximal to the olecranon along with tenderness and a positive Thompson squeeze sign (as for Achilles tendon rupture), where the arm is supported and the elbow flexed at 90°, may differentiate a partial rupture from a complete.

*Treatment.* Acute surgery with tendon suture and reinsertion of a bone flake is recommended for complete ruptures. However, nonsurgical treatment such as elastic bandage and a plaster splint would also be justified (especially at partial ruptures).

# Elbow Pain

## Overuse Injuries

### Radial Epicondylalgia (Tennis Elbow) * M77.1

*Diagnosis.* The most common elbow complaint and the most common enthesopathy (tendon insertion pain) of the entire body. On the whole, it is one of the most common conditions of the musculoskeletal system, both the prevalence and incidence of 1–2 % of the adult population. The highest incidence is seen in the age 40–50 span. The term "tennis elbow" is in fact somewhat dubious, or a misnomer, since the clinical patient group triggered by tennis playing only makes up for a very small part (although it is quite common for tennis players as such). Above all, the widespread and prevailing term lateral epicondyl*itis* is misleading since no inflammation, i.e. *-itis*, is proved except for the very initial phase. Surprisingly, the patients are often (up to 1/3 of the cases) unable to report any incidents of overexertion as the provoking cause. The condition affects people of both light and heavy labour. The diagnosis is made from the following: *(1)* a relatively typical history of radial elbow pain correlating to eccentric stress and loading, sometimes with a sudden, but generally gradual (70 %) onset, characteristically aggravated by (overhand) hard gripping and supination loading. Sometimes also presenting aching at rest in the worst cases; *(2)* tenderness at distinct palpation on the radial epicondyle of the humerus (see Fig. 1); *(3)* pain being provoked by *(a)* dorsal extension of the wrist with resistance (preferably with the elbow extended) and *(b)* Maudsley's middle finger test releasing pain at the elbow when the extended third finger is pressed down in the direction of the flexion.

Weakness may also be noted and finally *(4)* pain at the radial epicondyle when performing Mill's tennis elbow test, which is when the elbow is actively moved from flexion to full extension with the forearm in pronation and wrist in flexion (i.e. stretching position).

S.-A. Sölveborn, *Emergency Orthopedics*,
DOI 10.1007/978-3-642-41854-9_28, © Springer-Verlag Berlin Heidelberg 2014

**Fig. 1** Typical areas of
where tenderness is palpated
to differentiate radial
epicondylalgia ("tennis
elbow") from a radial nerve
entrapment: for the latter, the
thumb is placed
corresponding to about two
fingerbreadths distal to the
epicondyle, whereas the
tenderness experienced at
tennis elbow pain is most
apparent over the little groove
(sulcus) in the epicondyle
bone prominence

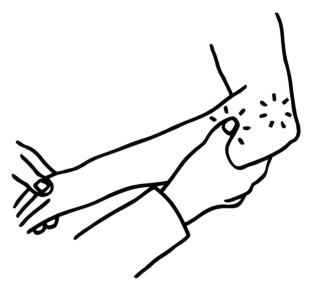

*Treatment.* *(1)* Initial treatment should include stretching with daily self-training exercises, 2–3 times a day, which is both inexpensive and free of side effects, and scientifically it has been proven successful (e.g. research results that have been published by the author; see Fig. 2). Other Swedish studies have pointed out that *(2)* eccentric wrist training may reduce the symptoms considerably in majority of the patients. As a complement, a so-called *(3)* "epicondylitis" forearm band may be used and empirically well proven is *(4)* local cortisone injections. One injection only may be enough, but then there is a significant risk of relapse within 3 months, thus, two injections are sometimes needed. However, the recommendation is to never administer more than three (at intervals of about 3 weeks). It is important that the needle is placed distinctly on the bone attachment of the radial ("lateral") epicondyle where the maximum tenderness is localised (generally this is immediately distal to the prominence of the radial epicondyle down the small sulcus at the enthesis of the extensor carpi radialis brevis – ECRB) and not too superficial, which may only result in a disturbing patch due to subcutaneous hypotrophy.

Research (mainly Swedish) supports the favourable effects of *(5)* deep acupuncture of classical type, as well as the more seldom accessible *(6)* ECSWT, extracorporeal shock wave therapy. Naturally, all patients should receive *(7)* ergonomic advice including instructions to take breaks, avoiding superfluous strain on the arm, such as overhand gripping, supination loading (e.g. screwdriving, stiff key locking) and hard handgrip manoeuvres (e.g. hammer work). At therapy-resistant cases of the nonsurgical options, *(8)* surgery may be indicated, and if so, one should not wait too long (preferably within 3–6 months) since it is now well known that the prognosis is better when surgery is performed at an earlier stage, contrary to what previously has been recommended. Research has shown that surgery according to the Hohmann

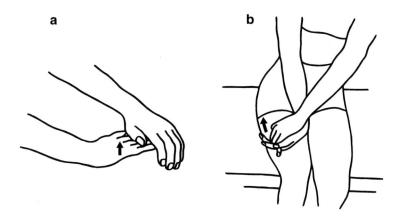

**Fig. 2** The stretching technique for radial epicondylalgia: (**a**) first, contraction of the forearm extensors with resistance for 6–10 s, then (**b**) immediately begin stretching with complete flexion and pronation of the relaxed hand (supported e.g. against the thigh) and traction of the fingers up towards the face. Maintain the position for 15–20 s, two to three sets twice a day

method with a release of the common extensor origin renders good or excellent results within the 77–94 % range. In general, there are in fact over 40 treatment methods described for "tennis elbow". In the acute phase, NSAID-gel may be tried, and possibly laser as well, and transverse manual friction therapy through referral to a physiotherapist.

## Ulnar Epicondylalgia (Golfer's Elbow) * M77.0

*Diagnosis.* Corresponding aetiology and histology as for radial epicondylalgia ("tennis elbow"). But golfer's elbow occurs only at about 20 % of the "tennis elbow" frequency; however, they sometimes occur simultaneously. This condition is also sometimes dubiously called "medial epicondylitis" and presents itself with pain at the ulnar ("medial") humerus epicondyle, sometimes also radiating down distally. The pain is accentuated at wrist flexion and pronation with resistance. Tenderness at palpation on the flexor/pronator origin and a notable association to ulnar nerve entrapment (in surgically treated groups in fact seen in 60 % of the cases).

*Treatment.* Active rest, loading modification, NSAID-gel initially and stretching of the flexors of the forearm. "Epicondylitis"/forearm band may be tried, and if the pain does not yield within 5–7 days, local cortisone injection may also render a good result when administered straight into the punctum maximum of the tender-ness. If so, be observant of the localisation of the ulnar nerve and give the injection preferably with the elbow extended. Physiotherapeutic measures are included in the treatment arsenal, and unyielding cases may be operated similarly to "tennis elbow" with flexor release and excision of fibrotic tissue. Often concomitant ulnar nerve decompression (neurolysis) must be performed depending on the symptom variation.

## Radial Nerve Entrapment, Radial Tunnel Syndrome * G56.3C

*Diagnosis.* Above all, this is a differential diagnosis to radial epicondylalgia ("tennis elbow"), but is concomitant to "tennis elbow" to a greater extent than was previously recognised, more than likely up to 15 % of the cases. Sometimes the radial tunnel syndrome is called supinator syndrome or *posterior interosseous nerve syndrome (PINS)*. Often an aching pain slightly distal to the elbow joint over the dorsal/radial area underneath the extensor muscle mass, often with radiating pain both distally and proximally. Tenderness at palpation of the radialis/supinator slit (see Fig. 1, page 190) down towards Frohse's arcade. The passage of the deep branch (interosseous posterior) of the radial nerve into the "radial tunnel" causes an entrapment. The latter may also in (very) rare occasions and occur at the upper arm due to a diaphyseal humerus fracture upon which the radial nerve is damaged. EMG/neurography seldom offers any additional facts to the diagnostics. Pain at supination with resistance.

*Treatment.* For non-traumatic cases symptomatic therapy, stretching, may be tried. At unyielding conditions, surgery with neurolysis of the radial nerve branch may be preferred.

## Ulnar Nerve Entrapment, Cubital Tunnel Syndrome * G56.2C

*Diagnosis.* The most common entrapment syndrome of the body after carpal tunnel syndrome. The nerve is compressed in the cubital tunnel in connection with the ulnar nerve sulcus, producing tenderness and pain at the "inner side" of the elbow along with paraesthesias and numbness (especially during night time) in the 4th and 5th fingers. Is generally aggravated by elbow flexion. Tinel's percussion sign is positive, in general, but EMG/neurography does not really contribute to the diagnostics (often negative initially). Sensory impairment of the little finger (most easily noticed at the two distal phalanges) and of the ulnar side of the ring finger (see Fig. 1 of chapter "Neck Pain", page 146).

*Treatment.* Activity adjustment and extension splint with merely a modest flexion for nocturnal use, possibly even at daytime for 3–4 weeks, may be tried, as well as flexor stretching. Unyielding, difficult cases may be operated on with ulnar neurolysis upon which a compression at the flexor notch of the nerve entrance, distal to sulcus, is most often found.

## Pronator Teres Syndrome G56.1C

*Diagnosis.* A median nerve compression at the passage through the pronator teres muscle at elbow level, which produces an aching pain around the elbow and proximally in the forearm corresponding to the flexor muscles. Weakness and discomfort, but usually no paraesthesias or sensory reduction of the hand. Tenderness at palpation and a positive Tinel's sign over the nerve at elbow level. Pain at pronation with resistance and occasionally at flexion of the middle finger (superficialis tendon).

*Treatment.* Adjustment of the workload, alternative training and surgery if not yielding.

## Synovitis–Arthritis, Synovial Impingement M02.9C/M07.3C/M11.8/9C/ /M65.9C

*Diagnosis.* Relatively uncommon. Occurs in all ages. It has a similar frequency rate for men as for women. Pain at movement, particularly at the end positions and mostly at extension. In the background there is trauma, overuse injuries and inflammatory joint disorders, where the latter may present joint swelling, which is felt most apparently laterally/radially (effusion around the "soft spot" of the lateral triangle: olecranon–epicondyle–caput radii). Sudden pain attacks can be explained by a synovial impingement. May lead to a certain degree of contracture. But a painful and limited range of motion occurs at an early stage.

*Treatment.* Activity adjustment, possibly NSAID-drugs in the very initial phase. Physiotherapy including strength and flexibility exercises is recommended. However, there is contraindication for forceful, aggressive, dynamic stretching of bouncing character and manipulation since there is an obvious risk of deterioration. Always avoid prolonged immobilisation of the elbow, never more than 3 weeks in adults! Always perform joint puncture with aspiration at swelling/effusion (see the chapter "Basic Injection Techniques"). At remaining or recurrent elbow synovitis, arthroscopic surgery including synovial resection could be indicated.

## Loose Body of the Elbow Joint (Osteochondrosis, Osteochondral Lesion) M24.0C

*Diagnosis.* A locking phenomenon and pseudolocking, hooking, of the elbow. Intermittent or persistent range of motion limitation, particularly an extension defect, when the cause is an underlying trauma, which has produced osteochondral fragments or osteoarthrosis (OA).

Swelling and joint effusion may arise, as well as pain at movement, especially at extension, but pronation–supination should also be examined. Radiography may overlook loose bodies of pure cartilage, thus an MRI may be needed, which may also be able to visualise an osteochondral defect (osteochondrosis dissecans, OCD). *Mb Panner* is characterised by a cartilage defect on the capitulum humeri in children, even without any trauma.

*Treatment.* Arthroscopic extraction

## Arthrosis (Osteoarthritis – OA) M19.0/1/2C

*Diagnosis.* Pain at carrying and limited range of motion, first noted in extended position, whereas pronation–supination will withstand. Degenerative changes are seen on X-ray, such as osteophyte formation and subchondral sclerosis. Inflammatory reaction of swelling and heat. Sudden attacks of pain. A crepitus sound at joint motion and pseudolocking, hooking, may occur. Risk of contracture progression and ankylosis.

*Treatment.* NSAID treatment by course (e.g. 10–15 days) at inflammatory reactions along with physiotherapeutic training. Joint puncture with aspiration at effusion. Arthroscopy or other surgery may be indicated.

## Olecranon Bursitis (Student's Elbow) * M70.2

*Diagnosis.* "Student's elbow" presents tenderness and swelling over the olecranon, often with fluctuation, and displaceable indurations, "lumps" or bits of "gravel", may be palpated in the bursa. These are fibrotic parts and synovial tissue, on occasions cartilage like. A quick progression of swelling may be due to a trauma or an infection, where the latter also presents local redness and heat.

*Treatment.* At fluctuation, puncture with aspiration is performed. At signs of infection: Drainage of the synovial fluid, culture and antibiotics accordingly. At serous fluid, a local corticosteroid injection of 1–2 ml may be administered, and an elastic bandage, possibly a bump-protecting brace. At repeated recurrences, surgery with bursectomy should be taken into consideration.

# Forearm Injuries

## Radius and Ulnar Shaft (Diaphyseal) Fracture * S52.4

*Diagnosis.* High- or low-energy injury, which is caused by either an indirect or direct trauma. Fractures of the radius and ulnar shaft often occur simultaneously (the so-called double-pipe), in traffic accidents quite often an open injury. The fractures are often displaced and unstable. Pain and local swelling, important to perform a peripheral examination (distal status) to rule out a neurovascular compromise! Radiography must include the elbow and wrist to be able to identify fractures of, e.g. Monteggia or Galeazzi.

*Treatment.* Closed reduction and plaster-of-cast may be precarious due to the antagonistic effect of the various muscle groups. Thus, open reduction or osteosynthesis with plate and screws is the rule in adults. If the fixation is stable, in fact no postoperative immobilisation with plaster is required; instead motion training may be introduced immediately, but with caution.

In *children,* displaced fractures have to be reduced under general anaesthesia. Often a breaking of the contralateral corticalis must be performed by continuing the reduction manoeuvre further towards the opposite side ("overreduction") to attain a satisfactory position and a favourable prognosis. Avoid rotational misalignment and angulation sideways (are insignificantly corrected during growth). Fractures of the upper third of the diaphysis are fixed in supination, of the middle third neutrally, and of the distal third are fixed in pronation – all from the perspective of the muscle traction force. A plaster splint is placed so that it covers both the elbow and wrist for 4–6 weeks. An X-ray control after 7–10 days and again after 3 weeks if the plaster splint is to be shortened. If the closed reduction is not satisfactory, osteosynthesis with intramedullary nailing is performed. Up to 15° of fracture angulation is considered acceptable for solely high plaster-of-cast treatment.

S.-A. Sölveborn, *Emergency Orthopedics,*
DOI 10.1007/978-3-642-41854-9_29, © Springer-Verlag Berlin Heidelberg 2014

## Greenstick Fracture (in Children) * S52.2/3/4/5/6/8

*Diagnosis.* Presented as a faulty angulated position of the diaphysis without a visible fracture line through the bone (incomplete fracture, the so-called greenstick). Generally caused by a fall during play, often causing severe pain.

*Treatment.* Angulation up to 15° is accepted for a sole treatment of plaster-of-cast. As for the rest, a closed reduction and a high plaster for 4 weeks are almost always sufficient, an X-ray control after 1 week. When the reduction is made, an "overreduction" is performed all the way through so that the intact contralateral corticalis is broken, or it may easily become subject to redisplacement.

## Isolated Diaphyseal Ulnar or Radial Fracture S52.2

*Diagnosis/Treatment.* An isolated fracture of only one of the forearm bones, mostly the ulnar diaphysis, due to a fending off-injury. At a slight displacement, it may be treated with a high plaster splint for 1 week whereupon it is replaced by a forearm orthosis. If the contact area of the fractured ends of the ulnar is good, and the angulation is less than 15°, the orthosis does not need to include the elbow. A long treatment time is applied: 10–14 weeks for an ulnar fracture, but as much as 16 weeks for an isolated radius fracture. An isolated fracture of greater displacement is fixed with plate and screws at open reduction.

## Monteggia Fracture S52.0 + S53.0

*Diagnosis.* Diaphyseal ulnar fracture (generally proximal) and a concomitant dislocation of the radial head (generally volar). Caused by a direct trauma or a fall, is rare but may render considerable residual symptoms, which all together signifies the importance of having X-rays taken that include both the wrist and the elbow. Note the possibility of an *Essex–Lopresti fracture*, which involves a fracture of the radial head with a concomitant dislocation of the distal radioulnar (DRU) joint. Severe pain of the forearm is experienced, substantial swelling over the elbow and a faulty position. The deep branches of the radial nerve may be damaged, thus, the extensor strength of the wrist must be assessed.

*Treatment.* Must be reduced, closed reduction may be attempted. However, generally surgery with open reduction of the ulnar fracture and plate osteosynthesis is necessary whereupon the radial head is often reduced automatically – if not, this needs to be reduced openly as well. At stable fixation no plaster is required, instead active motion training may be introduced immediately.

In *children,* closed reduction under general anaesthesia is almost always successful through longitudinal traction of the forearm in supination so that the ulnar fracture is reduced, then flexion to 90° and pressure on the radial head, which is so easily reduced – if not already in place. Plaster fixation of the elbow in a slightly greater angle than 90° of flexion for 4–6 weeks. A customary X-ray control after 1 week.

*Reversed Monteggia fracture* with a dorsal or lateral dislocation of the radial head is even more unusual. Is reduced through traction in the longitudinal direction and pressure against the radial head. Fixation of the arm is instead made in the extended position.

## Galeazzi Fracture S52.3 + S63.0

*Diagnosis.* An unusual type of forearm fracture in both adults and children, including a fracture at the junction of the middle and distal third of the radius in combination with a subluxation/dislocation of the distal radioulnar (DRU) joint rendering a displacement of ulnar head (generally of dorsal type). It is caused by a fall on the straight arm, but may also occur due to a direct blow. Tenderness over the fractured area and the wrist and laxity of the DRU joint may be palpated.

*Treatment.* Should be treated by open reduction and plate fixation whereupon the ulnar head generally is reduced automatically at the same time. On occasions, a pin fixation of the caput ulnae is required.

In *children*, a closed reduction may be performed, and a circular plaster, also covering the elbow area, may be applied at 90° of flexion and a certain degree of supination for the duration of up to 6 weeks of immobilisation. An X-ray control within 1 week.

# Part XII

# Wrist

# Wrist Injuries

## Distal Radius Fractures (Colles', Smith's and Barton's) * S52.5/6

*Diagnosis.* Coined "the most common fracture in the world" (possibly with the exception of vertebral compressions since half of those are asymptomatic). Distal radius fractures are divided in *osteoporotic* (women >50 years of age, men >60 years of age or people who are biologically older and/or inactive people) fractures caused by low-energy trauma or *non-osteoporotic* (women <50 years of age, men <60 years of age, or people who are biologically younger, and/or active people with great demands to function fully) fractures caused by high-energy trauma. These are classified in the following groups: *Colles'* fracture (the most common type) with a dorsal deviation of the distal fragment, often a concomitant fracture of the ulnar styloid process. In the most classic cases, a silver fork deformity or bayonet misalignment is seen: *Smith's* fracture with a volarly displaced distal fragment ("reversed Colles' fracture") and a less evident misalignment of the external profile and finally *Barton's* intra-articular fracture with a volar, often proximally shifted, fragment that produces a volar subluxation of the carpus. Reversed Barton's fracture implies a distal fragment that is instead dorsally displaced.

In general, these are caused by a fall on the outstretched hand or with the hand under the body. Pain at movement, tenderness at palpation, swelling and, in the typical cases, a visible displacement. Perform a peripheral neurovascular examination (distal status) – the median nerve function in particular. Be sure to inform the patient that a remaining misalignment often may occur, which will not, however, render any significant functional impairment.

*Treatment.* Thus, there is great value of offering the patient *adequate information* about the injury, the treatment and the follow-up procedure, as well as that therapy must be *active*. All patients should be given instructions to raise their arms to full overhead position 50 times a day, which significantly reduces the incidence of the serious complication of sympathetic reflex dystrophy or shoulder–hand–finger syndrome. Note that the ulna + position, i.e. the axial compression, is the most

S.-A. Sölveborn, *Emergency Orthopedics*,
DOI 10.1007/978-3-642-41854-9_30, © Springer-Verlag Berlin Heidelberg 2014

crucial factor for the treatment result! Surgery is indicated at such shortening of the fracture of 5 mm or more. Also an articular surface hitch of >1 mm in intra-articular fractures entails a substantial risk of joint complications and a worse functional result.

There is no need for ordinary Colles' fractures to be immobilised for more than 3 weeks. Published research studies show that there are no apparent differences in radiography, range of motion and handgrip strength compared to 5 weeks of immobilisation. However, instead it has proved to cause less pain and demonstrates a better estimated function at the follow-up for a 3-week plaster time. Similarly, it has been shown that fractures having only a slight displacement of a radial shortening of <2 mm and a dorsal angulation of <5° against the longitudinal axis of the radius, treatment with only an elastic bandage renders an equivalent radio-logical outcome, faster rehabilitation, better handgrip strength and is less, or equally, painful than a plaster-of-cast immobilisation.

When choosing treatment methods, great attention should be paid to the *general fitness, age and expected functional demands* of the patient. No "golden standard" has been established for treatments of distal radius fractures, and surprisingly few studies of sound scientific design have been made. However, a modern concept, which is scientifically tested and presented by the author, is based on radiological images (see Fig. 1), as follows:

*(1) Slightly displaced* radius fractures (an axial shortening of <2 mm and <5° dorsal angulation in relation to the perpendicular plane) are treated with an elastic bandage (preferably double wrapping) for 3 weeks. However, providing a plaster splint for the first week may be less pain inducive. *(2) Moderately displaced* radius fractures (an axial shortening of 2–5 mm or >5° dorsal angulation in relation to the perpendicular plane) are reduced (see Figs. 2 and 3) upon anaesthesia (generally local infiltration of 10 ml local anaesthesia injected in the hematoma of the fracture) and provided with a radius plaster splint near the "functional position" of the wrist (not, however, in a distinct volar flexion) to be remained for a total duration of 3 weeks. *(3) Severely displaced* radius fractures (where an axial shortening of ≥5 mm is the only determinant factor) must be operated on immediately and, if the operating room is quickly available, without any prior reduction attempts in the emergency room. Indication for surgery is greater in patients younger than 60 years of age, particularly at non-osteoporotic fractures in men, e.g. at an axial shortening of >2 mm and a dorsal angulation of >20°.

The surgical method of choice is usually external fixation and, if possible, "non-bridging", i.e. the fixation pins are placed only in the radius for full wrist mobility. Another option may be Kirschner pins + plaster. *(4) Intra-articular* fractures, as described above. However, surgery is necessary if there is a joint incongruence with a hitch of >1 mm remaining after a closed reduction has been performed.

X-ray controls, first after the initial reduction and fixation, and then 10 days post closed reduction. The latter, however, is only for patients who have been provided with a plaster-of-cast. Thus, it is not necessary for those who have been externally fixated or for those having only an elastic bandage. If a redisplacement leads to

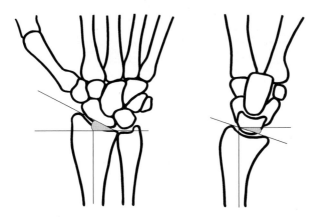

**Fig. 1** On the *left*: the wrist with angle markings for radial inclination from a frontal projection (normally on average 23°). *On the right*: the normal volar angle of the radius from a side projection (on average 12°). An axial shortening of the radius (clinically the most determinant measurement!) is usually established by measuring the distance between the ulnar edge of the radius and the plane joint surface of the ulna (so-called "ulna+"-value) from a frontal projection (*on the left*)

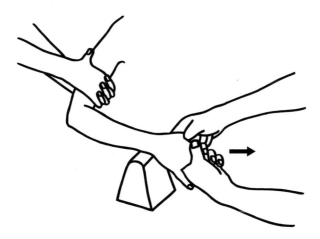

**Fig. 2** Reduction of a distal radial fracture in the classic way of pulling the thumb and the radial fingers while simultaneous counteraction is applied to the upper arm by an assistant, the wrist readily placed over a little wooden trestle

a nonacceptable position (ulna+ >4 mm, dorsal angulation of >20°), surgery should be performed. Possibly re-reduction and a new plaster-of-cast for a few cases with notably low functional demands. Generally, there is no gain in using radiography by routine at the final check-up and removal of the plaster.

N.B.! Be sure to inform the patients meticulously about the principle of treatment and expected result, preferably written information as well, handout written

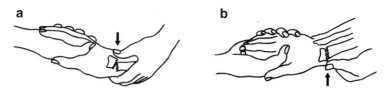

**Fig. 3** The distal fragment is then (**a**) pressed in place, and finally – if needed – (**b**) a correction of a radial translational displacement may be performed in a corresponding way from the side

motion training instructions for the fingers and the arm. In a great majority of the cases, an osteoporosis prevention and treatment programme should be implemented as well.

At *Smith's fracture,* a closed reduction with a pressure from the volar side should be performed. If a volar misalignment of <10° is present, a volar plaster splint is applied for 4 weeks, whereas *Smith* and *Barton* fractures with a volar misalignment of >10° are subject to surgery (with a volar support plate and postoperative immobilisation for 2 weeks).

A solitary *radial styloid process fracture* ("chauffeur's fracture") is treated with an elastic bandage if there is no sign of displacement, otherwise reduction under local anaesthesia and a plaster splint for 3 weeks. Note, however, that at a major displacement it may be associated with a (sub)luxation of the carpal bones (and a scapholunate dissociation).

Reduction manoeuvre (see Figs. 2 and 3, above) for distal radius fractures: Manual longitudinal traction of the hand/fingers, or by means of the Chinese finger trap, and counter-resistance applied to the upper arm having the elbow at a right angle. Keep the traction for a moment and then press your thumb against the distal fragment so that ad latus and angulation malpositions are corrected. A dorsoradial plaster splint of 12–15 cm is applied down to the finger knuckles whereupon the traction is gently released.

## Distal Radius and Ulna Fracture (including Physeal Damage) in Children S52.6

*Diagnosis.* Generally from fall on the outstretched arm and often during play. Represents half of all the physeal fractures. A typical dorsal displacement of the distal radial epiphysis along with a small metaphyseal fragment (Salter–Harris type II; see Fig. 2 of chapter "Ankle Injuries", page 42), which may be combined with a greenstick fracture of the ulna, a distal ulnar physeal fracture or a fracture through the tip of the ulnar styloid process. Fractures of Salter–Harris type III or IV with a displacement of the distal fragment are very rare.

*Treatment.* Infractions alone are stable fractures that require support only by a protective low plaster splint for 2–3 weeks, with no necessary X-ray follow-ups. Greenstick fractures with a moderate displacement are provided with a plaster splint for 3–4 weeks and a customary X-ray control 5–7 days post injury. Displaced fractures of >10–15° of angulation are reduced under general anaesthesia and may be troublesome. Traction alone is seldom enough but "hook-up" manoeuvres are required as well, e.g. an additional over-angulation of the fracture and applied pressure to the distal fragment so that the cortex on both sides of the fracture cling to each other whereupon the fracture may be straightened.

If the postreduction position is stable, a dorsal radius plaster splint is applied and kept on for 3 weeks, an X-ray control within 1 week. Open reduction is seldom required.

## Scaphoid Fracture * S62.0

*Diagnosis.* The most common fracture of the carpal bones, which particularly occurs in younger active men, such as athletes. Fall on the outstretched wrist and radially deviated hand, i.e. an indirect trauma to the scaphoid bone. The blood supply of the radial artery branches, which enter the bone distally and volarly, does not provide a favourable condition from a healing perspective for proximal and waist (midportion) fractures. All kinds of trauma, minor or major, may cause pain and weakness in the hand regardless of when in time the fracture occurred. Tenderness is presented in the fossa tabatière ("snuffbox") downwards between the EPL and APL tendons, especially at bi-digital palpation on both sides of the hand (see Fig. 4; note, however, that there may exist a slight tenderness in uninjured people as well), and when applying axial compression to the thumb and at forceful dorsal extension and radial deviation of the wrist. The fracture does sometimes not appear on the initial X-ray and for as long as 10–14 days post injury, but is visible on a scintigraphic bone scan within 2 days post injury, as well as on an MRI. If radiography is chosen, a new X-ray should be taken after 7–10 days, when a resorption zone is clearly seen.

*Treatment.* A scaphoid plaster-of-cast that extends over the midhand and down around the base phalange of the thumb. At clinical suspicion although presented by negative radiography, new X-rays are to be taken without the plaster after 7–10 days. Still being presented by negative X-rays despite severe tenderness, an MRI or a bone scan must be performed. A fracture should be assumed until tests prove otherwise. For proximal and waist fractures, the fixation time with plaster is 8–12 weeks. An X-ray control after 4 weeks.

A distal scaphoid fracture may then be left without plaster and be replaced by an elastic bandage for a short time. The rest are provided with a new plaster and a renewed X-ray control after 1 month. A fracture of >1 mm of displacement should

**Fig. 4** Palpation
(bi-digitally) of the scaphoid
bone at the "snuffbox"

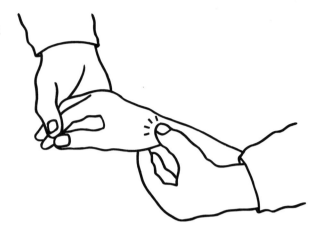

be considered for surgery and even a particularly more liberal indication in patients whose hands are subject to great loading, such as athletes. Fresh fractures with no greater misalignment, which have been treated with plaster, have a healing rate of 90 %. However, at pseudoarthrosis development (the proximal fracture types have the most negative prognosis), surgery is recommended already after 4 months. Pseudoarthrosis is worth performing surgery on even after several years.

## Scapholunate Dissociation S63.3

*Diagnosis.* In fact fairly common, but often overlooked, it is an interosseous ligament tear that renders a volar tilting of the scaphoid bone, which on a projection from the side exposes a zigzag position of the carpal bones, a so-called DISI pattern (dorsal intercalated segment instability) as well as a typical widening of the gap between the lunate and the proximal pole of the scaphoid at radiography of 2 mm, called the "Terry Thomas sign" (after the English actor with a gap between his front teeth, also known as David Letterman's sign).

Pain at movement and tenderness at palpation, but inconsiderable swelling. If untreated, there is great risk of arthrosis (OA) development. May be tricky even for radiologists to detect misalignments in the carpus.

*Treatment.* Anatomic reduction and ligament repair generally performed at a hand surgery unit. Fixation with pins may be necessary. Postoperative plaster for 6–8 weeks.

# Triquetral Fracture ("Dorsal Chip Fracture") S62.1

*Diagnosis.* Wrist pain after trauma. If an avulsion of a ligament attachment with a pulled bony fragment from the dorsal area of the carpus exists, it is more often from the os triquetrum. Tenderness at palpation dorsally and ulnarly with tiny swelling.

*Treatment.* Good blood supply presents favourable healing conditions, and 2 weeks of elastic bandage or plaster splint may be sufficient, no X-ray follow-up necessary. At severe displacement, open reduction should possibly be considered.

*Fractures of other carpal bones* in connection with a major injury should be assessed at a specialised clinic.

# Wrist Pain

## De Quervain's Disease (Tenosynovitis) * M65.4

*Diagnosis.* Stenosing tendovaginitis in the first dorsal tendon compartment with the abductor pollicis longus (APL) and extensor pollicis brevis (EPB) tendons affected may occur both with and without extra or unusual wrist exertion. Usually an intense aching pain over the radial styloid with local tenderness at palpation and swelling. Typically, it presents a positive Finkelstein's sign with induced pain through passive ulnar deviation of the wrist with the thumb flexed into the palm and the other fingers covering it (see Fig. 1).

*Treatment.* Often surgical, with cleavage of the first dorsoradial tendon compartment. However, a local corticosteroid injection into the tendon sheath may be tried, as well as a supporting wrist bandage for a few weeks. A locally applied NSAID-gel for some week is preferable to pills.

## Tenosynovitis Crepitans (of the Wrist Extensors) * M70.0

*Diagnosis.* Pain with a crepitus sound (tendon "creaking") on the dorsal side of the distal forearm radially, swelling and local tenderness with a "squeaking" sound upon palpation. Usually provoked by excessive dorsal extension movements of the wrist due to exertion at, for example, sorting and dividing of different things.

*Treatment.* Often an immediate effect from an intravenous injection of 15,000 IU heparin, which sometimes needs to be repeated after 1 day and possibly an additional time as well. Activity modification, stretching of the wrist extensors and locally applied NSAID-gel. Plaster splint is seldom necessary.

S.-A. Sölveborn, *Emergency Orthopedics*,
DOI 10.1007/978-3-642-41854-9_31, © Springer-Verlag Berlin Heidelberg 2014

**Fig. 1** The Finkelstein's test for Mb de Quervain of performing a passive distinct ulnar deviation of the wrist and the thumb fully flexed into the palm, tucked under the other fingers

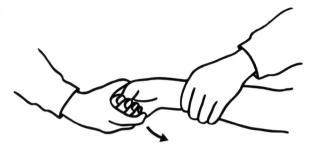

## Shoulder–Hand–Finger (SHF) Syndrome (Postfracture of Distal Radius), Reflex Sympathetic Dystrophy (RSD) T92.1/2

*Diagnosis.* Also called *finger–hand–shoulder (FHS) syndrome.* Aching pain, swelling and induration (organised oedema) of the hand and wrist along with limited range of motion in the hand, arm and shoulder. Usually autonomous nerve dysfunction as well with peripheral coldness, pale skin and sweating. However, initially warm, dry skin and burning and disproportional severe pain, which is worsened by palpation. May occur after a distal radius fracture and become chronic, but may also be caused by other injuries, even modest ones, or a hand operation. The aetiology is not fully established, but important factors are pain, anxiety and difficulty in initiating movements of the hand at an early stage of the healing process; all together a vicious circle is created. Patients often claim to have no use of the hand or arm at all.

*Treatment.* Intensified motion training supervised by a physiotherapist is of utmost importance since it may successfully break the vicious circle. Analgesics, elastic bandage and the arm elevated when there is swelling. At an established. FHS syndrome, a sympathetic block with local anaesthetics may both have a diagnostic and therapeutic effect in combination with occupational therapy and physiotherapeutic training. Daily exercise self-training programmes are important. TENS and acupuncture may be useful complements, and even antidepressants may be optional treatments.

## Wrist Ganglion M67.4D

*Diagnosis.* The most common soft tissue tumour of the hand and wrist. A cystic structure that emanates from the synovial membranes of a tendon sheath or the joint capsule (is then communicating with the wrist through a connection, i.e. a "stem" or "tube"), generally radially, and may occur both on the dorsal (most common) and the volar side. May be painful, tender at palpation, and produce symptoms due to the pressure. Contains a viscous, often very sluggish and jelly-like clear fluid.

The aching pain may be radiating, and it deteriorates at flexion or extension. Activity increases the size of the ganglion and may render limited range of motion.

*Treatment.* At acute symptoms, a short period of immobilisation may be alleviating, and the swelling may disappear spontaneously. The ganglion cyst should always be punctured and attempts to aspirate be made. The needle has to be thick considering the very viscous content, and there is an obvious risk of recurrence (30–50 %), even after surgical excision (5–10 %). A local corticosteroid may be administered at the time of puncture.

## Carpal Tunnel Syndrome (CTS) * G56.0

*Diagnosis.* Median nerve entrapment in the carpal tunnel (CTS), the most common compressive neuropathy. Seen predominantly in women (women/men ratio of 2:1) of 40–60 years of age (50 %) and may be particularly pronounced at the end of a pregnancy (most often released after the partus). An onset of nocturnal paraesthesias and numbness (due to a volar flexion position of the wrist during sleep) often beginning in the middle and ring finger, then a diffuse aching pain that may radiate to the thenar region, but also proximally up to the forearm.
The patients typically report of attempts to shake (or massage) the hand in the morning to "get the circulation back". Their night sleep is often also interrupted by the pain and numbness. At the advanced stage, constant problems with sensory disturbance, clumsiness of the hand, may be caused by straining or weight on the wrist in certain flexion. Even hypotrophy of the thenar muscles may occur. It may be a complication of a distal radius fracture (*do not* apply the plaster-of-cast in a distinct volar flexion for such a fracture).
   A positive Tinel's percussion sign is presented with paraesthesias of the median nerve distribution of the hand. A positive Phalen's volar provocation manoeuvre with numbness in the hand within 30 s (often 15 s or less) at forced flexion, preferably with the hand rotated towards the body. Weakness of thumb opposition may occur. EMG and neurography are not needed for the diagnostics, but may be resorted to when in doubt. Due to an anatomically more proximal anastomosis between the ulnar and median nerves, up to 30 % may also have symptoms in the two ulnar fingers.

*Treatment.* A stabilising, straight wrist splint, at least during night-time. Possibly a local corticosteroid injection, especially in rheumatic patients (has however a transient effect). For the most part, polyclinic carpal tunnel release surgery is needed.

## Ulnar Nerve Entrapment (in Guyon's Canal) G56.2D

*Diagnosis.* A rare nerve compression, usually due to a space-occupying process (ganglion, lipoma, aneurysm) or repetitive loading strain and local pressure from using tools, bicycle handlebars, etc.

Volar numbness and paraesthesias of the little finger and of the ulnar aspect of the ring finger, but seldom pain. Handgrip strength and thumb–index finger (pinching) grip may be weakened. A positive Tinel's sign at percussion over the ulnar Guyon's canal, the tunnel that runs between the pisiform bone and the hook of the hamate bone. EMG adds nothing to the diagnostics.

*Treatment.* Adjustment of weight load and strain on the hand and upholstered protection, possibly a wrist splint/wrist brace, but usually indication for surgery in persistent cases.

## Arthritis/Synovitis M02.9D/M07.3D/M11.8D/MM11.9D/M65.9D

*Diagnosis.* Wrist pain of degenerative, inflammatory and/or traumatic origin, also with distal radioulnar joint instability and arthrosis (OA). Swelling, stiffness and limited range of motion. At inflammatory arthritis, as in RA, tendon sheath swelling and synovial thickening as well. Sudden pain attacks likely pertaining to synovial impingement.

*Treatment.* Elastic bandage, contingent wrist puncture and aspiration and possibly a local corticosteroid injection, analgesics and short treatment course with NSAID.

## Stress Fracture of the Radius M84.3D

*Diagnosis.* A rare fatigue failure of the epiphysis/metaphysis of the radius after repetitive compressions and rotations of the wrist, almost always seen in younger athletes, such as gymnasts. Produces wrist pain, particularly radially–volarly, tenderness at volar and dorsal palpation of the distal radius.

*Treatment.* Active rest. Straining arm exercises should be avoided for 6–8 weeks.

# Hand Injuries

*Important to establish a meticulous patient's history: When? Where? How? Perform a peripheral neurovascular examination (distal status): Assess sensory functions radially and ulnarly, motility and peripheral pulses/skin tissue perfusion! Examine the separate functions of the profundus and superficialis tendons, as well as the extensor tendons. All of the above-mentioned examinations must be done **before** anaesthesia. For skin lesions: Cover up with remaining skin since the own skin is always the best dressing.*

## Scaphoid Fracture S62.0

See the chapter "Wrist Injuries".

## Scapholunate Dissociation ("Terry Thomas'/David Letterman's Sign": Ligament Injury, DISI) S63.3

See the chapter "Wrist Injuries".

## Triquetral Fracture ("Dorsal Chip Fracture") S62.1

See the chapter "Wrist Injuries".

## Hamate Fracture (Hamulus) S62.1

*Diagnosis.* Uncommon. But a fracture at the volar hook of the hamate bone, hamulus, may be associated with an ulnar nerve entrapment. Generally caused by a direct trauma to the volar, but also due to minor yet repetitive weight and strain

S.-A. Sölveborn, *Emergency Orthopedics*,
DOI 10.1007/978-3-642-41854-9_32, © Springer-Verlag Berlin Heidelberg 2014

injury, which subsequently will result in a stress fracture. Swelling, pain at wrist motion and tenderness at palpation ulnarly over the volar part of the hamate bone. However, it is not visible at ordinary radiography projection; instead a carpal tunnel view or CT is required.

*Treatment.* An ulnar wrist plaster splint that includes dig 3–5 is provided for 5 weeks, but often the hamulus requires surgical excision. Screw osteosynthesis may also be performed.

## Metacarpal Fractures * S62.3, S62.2

### Subcapitular (MC 5: Boxer's Fracture) S62.3

*Diagnosis.* A common fracture, which is caused by, e.g. a punch against a fixed object. Most often the neck of the 5th MC is affected. Often presents a volar displacement, a possible malrotation may be noted if the fingers are flexed (should point symmetrically to the scaphoid; see Fig. 3, page 219). The knuckle often becomes less prominent. Pain at movement, local swelling and tenderness at palpation, but seldom any sense of instability. A characteristic, indirect pain at axial compression of the finger.

*Treatment.* A volar fracture angulation up to 20° for dig 2 and dig 3, up to 30–40° for dig 4 and dig 5, may be accepted since this generally does not render any functional restriction. Closed reduction under local anaesthesia is performed by traction initially and then pressure to the fragment upwards from down below through a dorsal pressure direction of the finger when flexed at 90° at the MCP joint in combination with applied counterpressure just proximal to the fracture (see Fig. 1). A rotational displacement, however, is not accepted. A plaster-of-cast splint is then provided, which includes the adjacent finger for support for 3 weeks, fixing the MCP joints at 80–90° of flexion and the IP joints at 10° of flexion, to be replaced by a two-finger brace (tape or Velcro) for another 1–2 weeks in combination with introductory rehabilitation training. On few occasions, a pin fixation, or another osteosynthesis, is required if the position will not remain stable.

### Diaphyseal S62.2, S62.3

*Diagnosis.* Caused by either an indirect or direct trauma (such as a crush or squeeze injury). Be sure to note a possible rotational displacement (see Fig. 3, page 219). Usually a fracture of quite stable character.

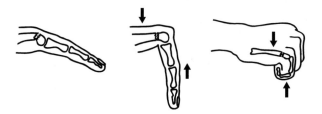

**Fig. 1** Reduction of a subcapital metacarpal fracture (usually MC 5) at 90° in the MCP joint and pressure in a dorsal direction away from the volar side while applying counteraction diaphyseally on the dorsum of the hand

*Treatment.* A slight shortening (of 2 mm) and volar angulation of 20° may be accepted; overlapping fractures are reduced. A volar plaster splint is provided for 3–4 weeks. Sometimes, e.g. for unstable, transverse fractures, surgery is required, then mostly through closed reduction and percutaneous fixation with pins. Plate fixation may be indicated on rare occasions. If the osteosynthesis is very stable, motion training could be introduced by an occupational therapist already 2–3 days postsurgery through the use of a removable orthosis. An X-ray control after 1 week and extraction of the pins 6–8 weeks postsurgery.

## Bennett's Fracture (MC 1 Base, CMC 1 Joint) S62.2

*Diagnosis.* An intra-articular fracture through the base of the first metacarpal that is displaced from its ulnar–proximal corner, where the volar lip fragment almost always remains in its ordinary place (strong ligament), while the metacarpal bone buckles radially–proximally and slightly dorsally (traction of the APL tendon; see Fig. 2). Usually caused by a direct blow to the pinching grip of the thumb–index finger. Instability of the CMC 1 joint. Pain at movement, local tenderness and swelling.

*Treatment.* Reduction to anatomic position is desirable and possibly; it may be done through closed reduction, but osteosynthetic surgery is preferable and routinely carried out through radioscopic percutaneous pinning (1–2 pins). Subsequently, immobilisation with a plaster splint for 5–6 weeks and a customary X-ray control after 1 week. Plaster and pins are to be removed after 6 weeks (no X-ray required), followed by motion training.

## Rolando's Fracture (MC 1 Base, Comminute or T-Fracture) S62.2

*Diagnosis.* A T-fracture through the base of the first metacarpal, but also the label for all comminuted intra-articular fractures of the thumb base.

*Treatment.* Open (or closed) reduction and pinning, then as described above for Bennett's fracture.

**Fig. 2** Bennett's fracture at
the base of the metacarpal of
the thumb, where the volar
joint fragment has remained
in its ordinary place while the
main fragment is posteriorly
proximally subluxed through
the traction from the APL
muscle

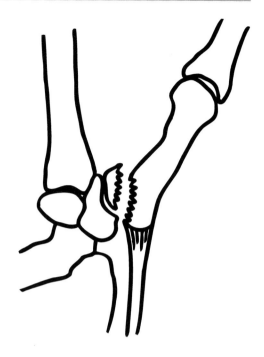

## Reversed Bennett's Fracture (MC 5 Base) S62.3

*Diagnosis.* An intra-articular fracture through the base of the fifth metacarpal, which is subluxated through traction of the ECU tendon in an ulnar–proximal direction, while the radial corner fragment still remains in its position. It is also called "tenneb fracture", i.e. Bennett spelt backwards.

*Treatment.* For this type of fracture, closed reduction has a greater chance of being successful than at the ordinary Bennett's fracture, but generally a radioscopic percutaneous pin fixation is required. A plaster splint is provided for 6 weeks whereupon it is removed at the same time as the pins.

**Fig. 3** A rotational misalignment must not be overlooked at finger fractures: the relative position of the finger nails at flexion in regard to their level and direction (shall point to the scaphoid) is helpful

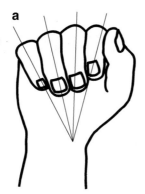
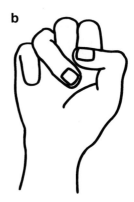

## Finger Fractures * S62.6 (Thumb S62.5)

### Middle and Proximal Phalangeal Fractures

*Diagnosis.* Caused by either direct or indirect trauma. Squeeze/crush injuries are common, where pertaining wound injuries and open fractures may occur as well. Swelling, deformity and tenderness, limited range of motion and pain at movement. May be considerably displaced due to traction of the tendons. A rotational misalignment must never be overlooked; radiography is, however, in this case, not optimal for an accurate description – look at the internal positions of the fingernails at flexion (see Fig. 3)! Also apply axial compression during the examination, i.e. pressure in the longitudinal direction (see Fig. 4).

*Treatment.* Reduction (see Fig. 4) under local anaesthesia/finger base block and then often fixation with a volar splint to be kept for 1–3 weeks whereupon mobilisation is introduced with a two-finger "buddy" splinting, i.e. two fingers taped together so that one acts as a splint/support, for an additional 2–3 weeks. The splint is arranged at 80–90° of flexion in the MCP joints and at 10° of flexion in the IP joints. For displaced and unstable fractures, particularly if a rotational misalignment remains, surgery with crossed pins may be necessary, preferably percutaneously. At undisplaced fractures, the finger may be taped to the adjacent finger, "buddy splinting", with upholstery in between the fingers, for 2–3 weeks and an X-ray control around the fifth day.

### Distal Phalangeal Fractures

*Diagnosis.* Easy to confirm with ordinary radiography. Special cases including children with physiolysis in the distal phalanx exist, which require immediate reduction.

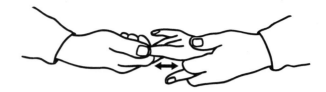

**Fig. 4** The position for reduction of a finger fracture (and dislocation), as well as for examination with axial/longitudinal compression ("indirect tenderness")

*Treatment.* Fractures of the processus unguicularis may be left untreated. However, proximal transverse fractures with a displacement require reduction, which generally is easily managed. At difficulty in maintaining the position, particularly if there is a large fragment including the joint surface, and/or volar subluxation, surgical fixation is on occasions performed with a percutaneously applied pin, which is removed after 3 weeks.

## Intra-articular Fractures

*Treatment.* Require exact reduction to render full joint congruity. A displaced fragment that involves more than 1/3 of the joint surface presents indication for closed, or open, reduction and osteosynthesis, generally with two obliquely applied pins. A volar fracture of an interphalangeal joint, a so-called Wilson's fracture, may, if it is more extensive, lead to a dorsal subluxation of the middle phalanx (whereas the volar fragment is often still in place) and requires a reduction and a pin fixation for 3 weeks. Only a small volar fragment in the PIP joint from the base of the middle phalanx may remain untreated.

## Finger (Phalanx) Dislocation (PIP, DIP) * S63.1

*Diagnosis.* Quite a common injury, particularly in ball sports. Generally, the little finger is affected in the PIP joint or the thumb through a side-to-side or hyperextension trauma. Swelling, tenderness and misalignment of the middle phalanx, usually in a dorsal and/or ulnar angulation position, which may either be slight or substantial with almost 90° of angulation. In half of the cases with such lesions of the collateral ligament, a small avulsion is seen on X-ray images, which are to be taken after the reduction is performed. The DIP joints and the IP joint of the thumb dislocate more seldom (if so, due to a hyperextension trauma), and a following inability to flex may be misinterpreted as a flexor tendon rupture.

*Treatment.* In general, immediate reduction is easily managed (sometimes even without any local anaesthesia) through traction (and gentle flexion) in the longitudinal direction of the affected finger (see Fig. 4). Postreduction radiography should always be performed. At distinct swelling and tenderness, an immobilisation for some week may be prescribed, otherwise direct mobilization with a two-finger "buddy splinting" for 3 weeks. This is applicable also for complete ligament injuries with side-to-side laxity. Be sure to inform the patient of local tenderness and swelling that may remain for quite a long time, as much as 6–12 months!

The finger needs to be protected during sports with a two-finger "buddy splinting" for a long time. Sometimes remnants of ligament fragments, or the "volar plate" (fibrocartilago volare), may be interponated (wedged) in the joint making it impossible to attain a correct position during closed reduction whereupon a surgical exploration needs to be done instead. At remnants of bone fragments of more than 1/3 of the joint surface, a closed or open reduction is also performed and transfixation with pin. Check the extension ability of the PIP joint after the reduction so that the attachment of the extensor tendon to the base of the middle phalanx has not been released.

## Metacarpophalangeal (MCP) Joint Dislocation S63.1

*Diagnosis.* Primarily seen in the MCP 1, secondly in the MCP 2. Often due to a hyperextension trauma. The patient is unable to flex the joint from the hyperextended position. Swelling and tenderness.

*Treatment.* A closed reduction of the MCP 1 is generally possible, whereas the MCP 2 often needs to be treated through open reduction due to the interposition/ wedging of soft tissue. In both cases, a plaster splint is provided for 2 weeks and then active movements are introduced.

## Finger Amputation (Fingertip Injuries, Partial/Total) S68.1 (Thumb:), S 68.0

*Treatment.* A fingertip injury where the bone is not exposed is dressed once every day to once every third day. A fingertip injury where the bone is exposed is treated by resection alone of a few millimetres of the distal phalanx. Open dressing with an ointment and saline compress, redressing after 5–7 days. An expected healing time of 3–4 weeks. Appropriate infection prophylaxis with penicillin for 3 days. Oblique fingertip amputations with a pertaining volar defect are treated with dressing only, whereas those with dorsal defects (as well as for amputations more proximally) are additionally taken care of through a shortening of the bone and subsequent suturing up of the volar skin. For a transverse amputation through the distal phalanx, a local V to Y skin plasty (according to Atasoy–Kleinert) may preserve the actual length of the finger.

Proximal amputation of the distal phalanx near the DIP joint is adjusted through exarticulation of the joint and closing of the defect with skin flaps of fish mouth-look upon a smoothening of the condyle on the middle phalanx. To avoid neuroma formation, the digital nerves are pulled forward and shortened by some cm or so. The nail matrix must be fully excised if a dorsal skin area is to be preserved and sutured.

For proximal amputations of the middle phalanx, what is left of the phalanx may be saved if an active flexion of the stump is possible; otherwise, an exarticulation of the PIP joint is preferable.

## Replantation Injuries

*Indications.* Amputation of several fingers, or proximally to the IP joint of the thumb, particularly proximal to the PIP joints, brings about a consideration of replantation providing that the amputated parts are relatively intact and have not been crushed. Contact should be taken with a hand surgery unit. Measures at single finger amputations should be discussed from case to case. Replantation should always be attempted at middle hand, wrist and forearm levels.

*Measures.* The separated finger (body part) is left untouched, wrapped in moist saline compresses and placed in a plastic bag, or a sterile surgical glove, which in turn is sealed in ice water (no direct contact with the amputated finger). Amputated fingers may withstand ischaemia for 24–30 h at cooling. A large impending bleeding wound must of course be attended to and stopped. However, forceps or ligature should not be used on blood vessels, instead a manual compression for about 5 min should be used, then compression bandage and elevation.

## Nail Injuries (Subungual Hematoma) * S67.0

*Diagnosis.* A squeeze injury, which may be very painful due to the increased pressure of a *subungual hematoma*.

*Treatment.* The bleeding is easily evacuated through the classical treatment of nail perforation with a red-hot end of a straightened paper clip without any anaesthesia. At a lacerated *nail bed injury*, the nail is carefully removed and the bed is repaired with fine absorbable suture. The removed nail should be reused as protection as a part of the wrapping.

**Fig. 5** Stability testing of the UCL of the thumb in the MCP 1 joint: lateral provocation (side-to-side) is performed both with the thumb straight and flexed at 20°, compare with the healthy thumb

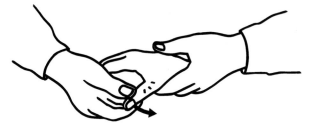

## UCL Tear ("Skier's Thumb") * S63.4

*Diagnosis.* Injuries of the MCP joint of the thumb are common, especially at skiing. A fall on the radially deviated (abducted) thumb is a typical cause. The ulnar collateral ligament (UCL) is generally ruptured distally and retracted proximally, whereupon the sharp proximal edge of the adductor aponeurosis may catch the torn ligament in a folded or rolled position, a so-called Stener's lesion. Pain at movement, swelling (bleeding) and tenderness at palpation over the ligament and down towards the volar side of the MCP 1 joint. Careful testing of the lateral stability (from side to side), both with the thumb straight and at 20° of flexion (see Fig. 5); compare with the uninjured thumb. Laxity at full extension indicates a complete rupture of the UCL. In case of a lateral instability, radiography should be performed.

*Treatment.* At an incomplete rupture with a distinct stop at the stability test may be treated with plaster-of-cast for at least 3 weeks. Tenderness and swelling may remain for 6–12 months! Sometimes the stability may be hard to assess and local anaesthesia with a digital block is required. At apparent laxity should surgery be executed, preferably by a hand surgeon polyclinically within a week. Postoperative plaster for 5–6 weeks.

Injuries to the *radial collateral ligament* are considerably more uncommon and should be treated with plaster for 4–5 weeks.

## Tendon Ruptures * S66.0/1/2/3/4/5/6/7

### Mallet Finger (Drop Finger) S66.3

*Diagnosis.* The most common extensor tendon injury, usually a flexion trauma against the extended finger, e.g. when a ball hits the tip of the finger and it "dips" down to a flexed DIP joint. A rupture of the extensor tendon occurs at the insertion at the base of the distal phalanx, but sometimes an avulsed fragment from the distal

**Fig. 6** Extension splint for
Mallet (drop) finger is fixed
with tape

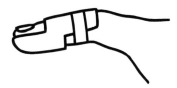

phalanx is seen on X-rays. Inability to fully straighten the fingertip actively, but full passive extension is possible. Tenderness and slight swelling.

*Treatment.* A plastic (or metallic) prefabricated extension splint, such as the stack splint (see Fig. 6), is applied at the DIP joint – it must not involve the PIP or MCP joints – to have day and night for 6–8 weeks and then as a night splint for another few weeks. At a greater, and displaced (>2 mm), avulsed fragment of more than 1/3 of the joint surface, and/or a subluxation of the distal phalanx, there is indication for surgery within a few days and transfixation of the joint (for 3 weeks). When necessary, a fixation of the bone fragment is done through pinning or with suture. Drop finger lesions older than several weeks (or even months) may also be successfully treated with the above described extension orthosis.

## Boutonnière (Buttonhole) Deformity M20.0

*Diagnosis.* A more uncommon lesion, which is caused by a flexion trauma to the PIP joint during active extension or from cutting. There is a rupture of the central band of the extensor tendon at the insertion of the base of the middle phalanx. The extensor mechanism is changed due to volar subluxation of the lateral bands of the extensor, whereupon they form a "buttonhole" for the condyle of the proximal phalanx and render a flexor function of the PIP joint. An untreated injury leads to the characteristic deformity with a flexion contracture in the PIP joint and a hyperextension misalignment of the DIP joint. Inability to actively and fully extend the PIP joint.

*Treatment.* Closed injuries are treated with an extension splint for the PIP joint and the DIP joint left free for 3–4 weeks. A transfixation of the joint with a pin percutaneously may be done as well. Open injuries, however, should be operated on with a similar pinning or a reinsertion in the event of a bone avulsion. After the immobilisation period, a dynamic extension splint is applied for another 2–3 weeks, hence permitting an active flexion of the PIP joint.

## Other Extensor Tendon Injuries S66.2/3

*Diagnosis.* Most extensor tendon injuries are generally sharp lesions caused by cutting incidents, for example. They occur on the fingers and distally at the hand's

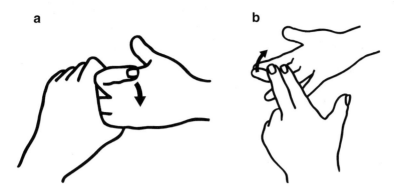

**Fig. 7** Function testing of the flexor tendons: the superficialis (sublimis) is tested by keeping the other fingers in full extension (**a**), the profundus by holding the PIP joint of the finger straight (**b**) whereupon the patient is asked to bend the injured finger

dorsal side, usually with only a slight retraction of a few mm of the proximal tendon part, whereas when occurring at the proximal region, the retraction may be greater, generally through the retinaculum of the wrist. The EPL tendon may spontaneously rupture, often at the tubercle of Lister, several weeks after a distal radial fracture as well as in rheumatics.

*Treatment.* Extensor tendons are sutured with 4-0 mattress sutures, or 3-0 more proximally, and the hand is immobilised with the wrist in dorsal extension of 45–60° and the MCP and PIP joints only slightly flexed. Pay careful attention to the risk of infection when the injury is caused by human bites on the tendons where antibiotic treatment is appropriate. The EPL is managed by hand surgeons through tendon transfer of the EIP or suture.

## Flexor Tendons Ruptures (Profundus/Superficialis) S66.0/1/6

*Diagnosis.* These are rather unusual injuries, which almost always occur in connection with wound injuries. The profundus tendon (or the FPL of the thumb), however, may rupture due to an extension trauma against a flexed DIP joint. The profundus tendon inserts at the distal phalanx while the superficialis tendon inserts at the middle phalanx. A functional examination to separate the two is performed by holding the other fingers locked in extension, and the affected finger may then be flexed in the PIP joint involving only the superficialis tendon (FDS, see Fig. 7a). The profundus tendon (FDP) is tested with the finger locked in extension at the PIP joint (see Fig. 7b). Radiography demonstrates any possible avulsed fragment. Zoning is applied to describe the level of the laceration, going from zone I, which includes the distal parts of the fingers, to zone V, which is proximal to the wrist. Zone II, with the area of the tendon sheaths (reinforced with fibrous bands at certain levels, the so-called annular ligaments, "pulleys") at the MCP joints and the adjacent distal area, is classically called the "no man's land".

*Treatment.* Always referral to a hand surgery unit for surgery. Antibiotics are prescribed if the wound is contaminated.

## Finger Distorsions (Joint Capsule Injuries) * S63.6

*Diagnosis.* Very common sprains, which usually are caused by a direct trauma to the finger by a ball, a fall or a "jammed" finger (the finger is caught in something). Finger swelling and pain, tenderness at palpation and limited range of motion (particularly at flexion) occur as a consequence of a joint capsule injury and partial tears of the collateral ligaments. Present adequate stability at laxity testing and an intact flexion and extension function. Normal radiography.

*Treatment.* Elastic bandage and a two-finger "buddy splinting". Taping (with an interposed compress) to the adjacent finger when resuming sports or other straining activities, which may be done as soon as and to an extent that the pain is tolerated. Note that normal range of motion, especially the flexion, almost always takes a long time to be restored after having had a PIP joint distorsion, and the finger may be swollen and stiff for 6–12 months.

## High-Velocity Injection Injuries W41

*Diagnosis.* The thin jet beam of a paint gun may have perforated the skin, and a highly tissue-toxic substance, such as paint, oil, solvent and antirust agents, disseminates widely and deeply at high pressure. The lesion may look innocent with only a tiny, visible entry, and there are initially little symptoms, but within a few hours large necroses may develop and fingers may be lost.

*Treatment.* Urgent transport to a hand surgery unit for emergency exploration and complete removal of the high-velocity injected substance, which may lead to extensive debridement and time-consuming surgery. Thus, it is always wrong to just wait and see!

# Hand Infections

## Paronychia * L03.0

*Diagnosis.* A common infection of all ages around the margins of the nail – the nail folds. It may form an abscess and also be spread under the nail. Redness, heat and swelling with pain along the margins of the nail are experienced. May be associated with nail-biting, manicure, hangnail or ingrown nail. Typical cases caused by *Staphylococcus aureus*.

*Treatment.* Elevation, immobilisation and antibiotics (flucloxacilline or cloxacilline are appropriate drugs of choice). At abscess formation, an incision is done parallel to the nail under local anaesthesia, a digital block. Subsequent culture and then left open without suture. At massive maceration, a resection of the lateral part of the nail (wedge excision) is required, possibly even a total avulsion.

## Panaritium (Infection of the Finger Pulp, Felon) L02.4

*Diagnosis.* An intracutaneous or subcutaneous infections of the finger pulp that may spread deeply and lead to a stud-like abscess with a wider deep lying part. If left untreated it may lead to tissue necrosis. The infection may even reach deeper and into the bone and develop a bone felon, osseous panaritium.

*Treatment.* Surgical drainage under digital block. At deep infection the incision is made longitudinally from the side of the finger. Antibiotics prescribed as for a paronychia, described above.

S.-A. Sölveborn, *Emergency Orthopedics*,
DOI 10.1007/978-3-642-41854-9_33, © Springer-Verlag Berlin Heidelberg 2014

## Septic Tendovaginitis/Tenosynovitis M65.0/1

*Diagnosis.* Tendon sheath infections may be caused by puncture wounds to the fingers, dog or cat bites, etc., but sometimes there is no evident explanation. The flexor tendon sheaths of dig 2, 3 and 4 are isolated, but those of dig 1 and 5 are communicating, which is why a so-called *V-phlegmon* may arise due to tendovaginitis of the thumb or the little finger. There are characteristic (Kanavel's cardinal signs) redness, swelling and tenderness corresponding to the flexor tendon sheath, as well as pain at active flexion, but particularly intense pain at passive extension. The finger is kept slightly flexed at rest. Often concomitant fever, lymphangitis and lymphadenitis. A confounding collateral oedema may be noted on the dorsal side of the finger or hand. Risk of rapidly necrotising flexor tendon.

*Treatment.* Immobilisation of the entire hand, elevation and antibiotics. Often an urgent need for surgical drainage, subsequent culture and tendon sheath lavage with large quantities of saline solution through incisions of its proximal and distal parts. Antibiotics, initially through parenteral administration, then a course of oral drugs, preferably flucloxacilline, cloxacilline or cephalosporin. Mobilisation with caution 3 days postsurgery – active motion training is important to avoid adherence formation.

## Volar Phlegmon M65.0, L02.4

*Diagnosis.* A deeply disseminated infection of the uncompact tissues distal to the palmer flexor crease, which may easily occur and render the fingers slightly abducted. In depth, there are radial and ulnar bursae, which are divided by a septum originating from MC 3.

*Treatment.* Abscess drainage with incisions both at the volar and dorsal side.

## Dorsal Phlegmon of the Hand L02.4

*Diagnosis.* A dissemination of a subcutaneous infection of the back of the hand. May produce extensive maceration.

*Treatment.* Drainage by one or several longitudinal slightly curved incisions over the back of the hand, whereupon a quick healing is generally rendered.

# Numbness in the Hand/Nerve Lesions

## Entrapment of the Median Nerve, Carpal Tunnel Syndrome * G56.0

See the chapter "Wrist Pain".

## Ulnar Nerve Compression * G56.2D

See the chapter "Wrist Pain".

## Cervical Rhizopathy, Herniated Disc M53.1, M50.1

See the chapter "Neck Pain".

## Nerve Cut Injury S64.0/1/2/3/4

*Diagnosis.* The sensibility is best tested by pinching with tweezers and not by pinpricking the sensory areas of the affected nerves (see Fig. 1 of chapter "Neck Pain", page 146). The sudomotor function disappears in denervated areas, which is why these sections become completely dried up. Loss of motor function is easily checked through thumb opposition (i.e. the combination of flexion and adduction) for the *median nerve*, through ab- and adduction of the fingers for the *ulnar nerve,* and by checking the extensor function of the MCP joints and the wrist for the *radial nerve.*

*Treatment.* Nerve injuries of the palm or forearm result in significant loss of hand function and should always be referred to a hand surgery unit for primary care.

S.-A. Sölveborn, *Emergency Orthopedics,*
DOI 10.1007/978-3-642-41854-9_34, © Springer-Verlag Berlin Heidelberg 2014

In essence, all sharp lacerations/cuts should be restored through suturing. Digital nerve lesions distal to the PIP joint caused by sharp cuts may be adapted upon suturing of the skin, or they should be attended to at an orthopaedic unit. However, the radial digital nerve of the index finger and the ulnar digital nerve of the thumb, which are of utmost importance, e.g. for the pinching and key grip, as well as more proximal nerve lesions, must be taken care of by a hand surgeon. At digital nerve sutures, a plaster splint is provided for 2–3 weeks.

# Part XIV

# Miscellaneous

# Burns T22/23/24/25/(20)

*An assessment of the burn surface is made according to the burn percentage rule of 9s, but it is easier to relate to the entire surface of the hand on the palmar side which is equal to 1 % of the entire body surface. Establish the history of the patient: When? Where? How? During the first 4 h after a (even a large) burn injury, the patient is relatively unaffected.*

*1st Degree.* Erythema with redness and a strong vascular dilatation, swelling and local pain.

*Treatment.* No specific treatment, but cooling liniment for pain relief.

*2nd Degree.* Caused by exposure to hot liquids, flames, steam, etc. and results in superficial, exudate-filled blisters, vesicles and often a considerable subcutaneous oedema. At *superficial* injuries there are "islands" of epidermis left and the healing is good, often leaving no scar formation. At *deep* tissue injuries leaving little or none of the epidermis, the healing is slower and renders scar formation (cicatrisation).

*Treatment.* Immediate rinsing and irrigation with cool (running) water – water-water-water! However, do not use water that is too cold and *never* use pieces of ice on a burn injury! Remove the clothes and shower for 20 min. Dressing, e.g. with a well-absorbent wringed-out saline compress, Jelonet or Aquacel bandage. Infection prophylaxis should be administered. Motion training, but with caution, is possible, particularly if a moist chamber, such as a plastic glove or a plastic bag, is used (which is to be changed every 3 h), or a sterile bandage, which is changed when soaked through. Do the wrapping crosswise to avoid the bandage from sagging.
For *children* it is advisable to use lidocaine and sodium bicarbonate moistened compresses. Analgesics, e.g. paracetamol, should be prescribed and possibly laughing gas for inhalation.

S.-A. Sölveborn, *Emergency Orthopedics,*
DOI 10.1007/978-3-642-41854-9_35, © Springer-Verlag Berlin Heidelberg 2014

*3rd Degree.* Caused by close encounters with open fire, very hot fluids or corrosive chemicals as well as electrical burn injuries. The entire layer of dermis is necrotising, may even include the subcutaneous and deeper layers. Substantial oedema is present, may be masked, however, by hard necrotic skin. At extensive injuries of the extremities, there is a risk of compartment syndrome or vascular strangulation.

*Treatment.* As a rule, the patient should be admitted to hospital. Prompt excision of necrosis. The defect should be covered through split-thickness (partial-thickness) free skin grafting or possibly through pedicle grafts. At extensive injuries and circular such: Skin decompression (through relieving incisions) and possibly fasciotomy. Intravenous infusion should be administered at burns of 10 % or more, preferably with Ringer's acetate the first day. Tetanus prophylaxis. Wash burned skin with liquid soap.

Referral to a *burn injury unit* for injuries of the 2nd degree including >20 % of the body surface in adults and >10 % in children and for patients older than 50 years of age. This applies to 3rd degree injuries of >5 %, particularly if the neck, face, hands, feet, genitals, perineum and joints are affected, and for electrical and chemical burns as well.

At acid burns: Rinse with water only! Basic injuries (e.g. caustic soda) are treacherous since deeper injuries gradually develop in a day or 2 – rinse (with water only) for a 24 h period!

# Basic Injection Techniques

## General Information on Joint Puncture

*Infection prevention is the key to successful surgical orthopaedic measures overall. It is imperative that joint puncture is performed at sterile conditions with adequate cleansing technique (begin where the needle shall be placed and clean outwards in a spiral fashion), fenestrated drapes, sterile gloves, hair protection (actually more important than a mouth mask, which in fact is not compulsory as long as one keeps quiet and does not cough or sneeze), 18–20 gauge needle (large enough to be able to withdraw viscous joint fluid) and 10 cc syringe* (e.g. *20 cc for knees, see* Fig. 6 of chapter "Knee Injuries", page 72). *Local anaesthesia is in fact not needed in general – involves only more pricking and thus more pain.*

*Mark the injection site with your nail or a pen. Always aspirate before an injection (note also the empty syringe prior to the injection). Ask if the patient suffers from any allergies. After an injection, do not leave the patient unattended. If possible, avoid injections in children – there is a risk of stigmatisation.*

## Knee Joint Puncture TNG10

"ALL KNEES WITH EFFUSION MUST BE PUNCTURED", mainly due to three reasons: (1) For the *diagnosis* (since joint aspiration reveals blood, a clear synovial fluid, a purulent or nontransparent punctuate, or fat pearls on the surface) and (2) for *symptom relief*, there is almost always an immediate good effect and that it is (3) *counteractive to quadriceps inhibition*, which is a complicating factor at joint effusion and/or joint pain.

The patient should be placed in prone position with the affected leg straightened and the quadriceps muscles relaxed (no cushion under the knee, which only constricts the joint space in the direction of the injection). Insert the needle just posterior to the upper lateral pool of the patella (see Fig. 3 of chapter "Knee Injuries", page 68, and

S.-A. Sölveborn, *Emergency Orthopedics*,
DOI 10.1007/978-3-642-41854-9_36, © Springer-Verlag Berlin Heidelberg 2014

Fig. 6 of chapter "Knee Injuries", page 72) somewhat obliquely, upwards–inwards, slightly proximal to the edge of the patella.

Use the other hand to, from a proximal position of the suprapatellar pouch, press down the joint effusion distally (a "bulge sign", see Fig. 2 of chapter "Knee Injuries", page 68), and/or the patella may be pressed carefully from the medial side to produce an angle for a wider insertion area.

If a positive "apicitis sign" (a.m. Puddu) is presented, an injection of a 1 cc combination of corticosteroid and local anaesthetics is administered obliquely up and into the inferior part of the distal patella pool using a rather long intramuscular needle from the distal side. At same time, pressure should be applied to the patella (as at the apicitis sign test) proximally so that the apex of the patella is slightly angled forwards. This injection for *jumper's knee* is administered for the purpose of collagen degradation to reduce adherences and fibrosis in the region of the proximal attachment of the patella tendon adjacent to the pain-inducing synovial fat pad of Hoffa.

## Shoulder Injections TNB10, TNB11

*Impingement test:* Inject local anaesthetics (10/cc/for the big ones and 5 for the small ones!) straight into the lateral (or anterior) side of the acromion with, as a suggestion, a long intramuscular needle that is aimed obliquely up and towards the inferior part of the acromion and the AC joint (see Fig. 3 of chapter "Shoulder Pain", page 166). Almost no resistance should be felt during the instillation. Wait for 15 min and repeat the impingement sign (e.g. according to Hawkins–Kennedy at 90° of abduction and inward rotation of the arm (downwards) at a slight flexion of the shoulder). The test is positive if a pain reduction of 80 % is assessed, a substantial improvement of the range of motion is generally attained as well.

*Rotator cuff syndrome with tenderness at the attachment of the subscapularis:* An injection that consists of a 1 cc combination of corticosteroid and local anaesthetics at punctum maximum of the humeral head into the tuberculum minus area anteriorly.

*Injection of the glenohumeral joint* may be administered either posteriorly or anteriorly – the latter seems to be the easiest and most obvious alternative – with the insertion placed in between the processus coracoideus and the humeral head.

*The acromioclavicular joint* is advisably reached from up above with a relatively thin needle, since it is a narrow joint, and generally only a maximum of 1 cc may be instilled.

## Elbow Injections

*Joint puncture* (TNC10) is performed in the "soft spot" slightly below the radial epicondyle just radial to the olecranon with a slight flexion of the elbow (see Fig. 5 of chapter "Elbow Injuries", page 185). An aspiration of a hematoma in the joint is recommended, e.g. for caput radii fractures to relieve the pain and to restore range of motion.

*Radial epicondylalgia:* An injection that consists of a 1 cc combination of corticosteroid and local anaesthetics is administered with a thin needle directly to the bone in the little groove (sulcus) where a relatively great resistance is felt during the instillation. Thus, the needle's attachment to the syringe should be squeezed to prevent it from coming off and causing a leakage. Place the arm at elbow flexion of at least 90°.

*Ulnar epicondylalgia:* As to a radial epicondylalgia corresponding injection that consists of a 1 cc combination of corticosteroid and local anaesthetics is administered directly to the ulnar epicondyle with a thin needle. Attention should be paid to the ulnar nerve of the cubital tunnel.

*Olecranon bursitis:* Perform a posterior puncture with aspiration of the cyst, and at noninfectious prolonged, or recurrent, bursitis a deposition of 1–2 cc of a corticosteroid may be administered as well. An elastic bandage is provided.

## Ankle Puncture TNH10

Advisably, to be performed through an anterolateral or anteromedial entry (see Fig. 1 of chapter "Ankle Pain", page 46) upon careful palpation, which starts at the corresponding malleolus and proceeds inwards anteriorly. Avoid the superficial fibular/peroneal nerve laterally and the vena saphena magna medially.

## Digital Block (of Foot and Hand)

Local anaesthetics of 6–10 cc without adrenaline are administered at the base of the toe or finger through a thin needle that is inserted on each side at the digital base at the metatarsal and metacarpal head level, respectively, into the web space alongside the extensor tendons from the dorsal surface. Preferably, a proximally placed rubber strap with a hemostatic forceps should be used for stasis, then wait for 10 min.

## Heel Injection

To be administered to the calcaneal insertion site of the plantar fascia. A 1 cc combination of corticosteroid and local anaesthetics may be injected at punctum maximum, possibly by injecting it obliquely from the medial plantar area.

## Hip Injections

*Trochanter major bursitis/periostalgia* is often injected with a 1 cc combination of corticosteroid and local anaesthetics laterally straight into punctum maximum of the bone with a long ("green") intramuscular needle.

*Joint puncture* (TNF11) of the hip is seldom indicated. Is then performed through radioscopy, generally with an anterolateral approach.

# Osteoporosis

M80.0, M80.2, M81.0, M81.2, M81.9, etc.

*Osteoporosis and fragility fractures are public health problems of great magnitude (possibly even the greatest of the Western world, although not fully recognised as such). Osteoporosis is a progressive and dangerous disorder, sometimes called the silent killer, e.g. hip fractures have a mortality of 20 % the first year after the fracture (32 % the second year)! Osteoporosis is generally detected when a fracture (the first) is presented. However, as much as 60 % of the vertebral compression fractures are asymptomatic. So far, the vast majority of patients having consulted a physician due to osteoporotic fractures did not have the classification code of osteoporosis registered in their medical chart (e.g. M80.0, M81.9).*

*Osteoporosis is best defined as a systemic bone disease with reduced strength due to decreased bone mass and/or bone quality with disturbed micro-architecture rendering an increased susceptibility to fractures.*

## Diagnostic Criteria

The definition of osteoporosis, according to the WHO 1994, is based on bone density measurements in younger women with a bone mineral density (BMD) of a 2.5 standard deviation (SD) from the average (i.e. the T-score) or more. *Severe (manifest, established) osteoporosis* includes not only this definition but an additional incident of fragility fracture is required as well. However, treatment (= prevention) may be safely initiated without a bone density measurement but based on the clinical picture alone. It should, in fact, be done so accordingly due to the following diagnostic criteria as incentives: *Old biological age; low-energy fracture/fragility fracture in patients older than 50 years of age of the types, (1) vertebral compression, (2) wrist fracture (distal radius), (3) hip fracture and (4) proximal humeral fracture (collum chirurgicum); in women of older age (particularly >70 years of age) and where a falling tendency is suspected and perioral corticosteroid medication for >3 months.* At the presence of one of the above-mentioned fragility fractures + old biological

S.-A. Sölveborn, *Emergency Orthopedics*,
DOI 10.1007/978-3-642-41854-9_37, © Springer-Verlag Berlin Heidelberg 2014

age, bone density measurement is thus not necessary in order to start the osteoporosis treatment! A history of a *previous fracture* is the strongest predictor of a recurrent fracture, and particularly vertebral compression is basically equivalent to an osteoporosis diagnosis! Other important risk factors that strengthen the indication for treatment are *low physical activity, low BMI (<19–20), early menopause (<45 years), mother who suffered from hip fracture and/or multiple vertebral fractures and alcohol abuse.* An X-ray interpretation that reports a "demineralised skeleton", bone loss or "picture framing" also serves as good indication for initiation of measures pertaining to osteoporosis. Radiography should in fact always be performed for patients >50–60 years of age who consult a physician due to (low) back pain for over 2–3 weeks. Osteoporosis must also be considered – in addition to the above-mentioned fragility and low-energy fractures (caused by a same-level fall) – at pubic ramus fractures of the pelvic ring and at certain ankle and knee fractures (e.g. in the tibial condyle).

## Patient Information

At indication of osteoporosis, information consisting of general advice and self-training exercises as proactive and preventive measures should be given to the patients, e.g. according to the easy-to-do and safe training programme shown here in Fig. 1. A supplementary questionnaire on risk factors should also be handed out, including instructions to contact their general practitioner for further measures and/or, when appropriate, a special osteoporosis clinic. The responsibility to investigate is definitely due when the patient has suffered from two osteoporotic fractures or one previous fracture + risk factor(s). An Internet-based instrument called FRAX (WHO: Fracture Risk Assessment Tool) is available for the calculation of the percentage risk of getting an osteoporosis-related fracture as well as a hip fracture within the next 10 years. The online tool is easy to use: www.shef.ac.uk/FRAX/.

*Treatment.* Is equivalent to *fracture prevention* and shall include these seven elements: (1) *Physical activity* – advice to exercise (load training) regularly, on a daily basis, for at least 30 min, proactive/preventive training (see Fig. 1). Possibly, referral to a physiotherapist with a prepared programme. (2) *Being outdoors* for sun exposure for 15 min a day. (3) *Quit smoking.* (4) A *diet* including 800–1,500 mg calcium (oral intake), e.g. dairy products (a glass of milk contains about 200 mg calcium, a slice of cheese 80 mg), soya and vegetables, and 10–20 μg vitamin D (400–800 IE), e.g. in oily/fatty fish and egg. (5) *Fall prevention* regarding risks in one's surroundings, such as rugs lying loose and electrical cords, imbalance and impaired vision to be compensated, and drug-induced dizziness. (6) A *preventive shock-absorbing hip brace, and a special corset for back conditions,* and finally (7) *medication* – the following alternatives are available: (a) vitamin D3 + calcium in a combination tablet, may even be administered to "all" patients >75 years of age

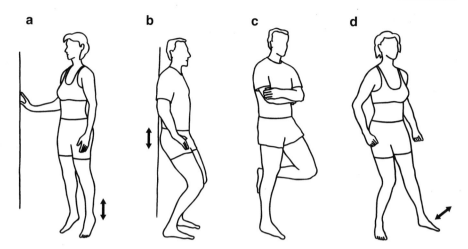

**Fig. 1** Exercises to prevent and counteract osteoporosis as well as the risk of fragility fractures:
(**a**) Heel-raises with hand support, 15–20 times, a progression may be reached through training of one foot at a time.
(**b**) Knee bending from standing position to 90° of flexion, 5–10 times, back support to a wall.
(**c**) Balance exercise with one-leg standing, preferably for 2 min, progression through eye-closing, then on more soft ground surface (e.g. blankets), and finally wobble board.
(**d**) Lunges; where the foot is moved to the side – from standing straight – and the weight being transferred to it, and back again. To be repeated in the same way – from standing straight – to the front, and then to the back, altogether (both feet) for 12–24 times

(!); (b) bisphosphonates (e.g. oral alendronate 10 mg × 1, or 70 mg once a week, risedronate 5 mg × 1, or 35 mg once a week, ibandronate 150 mg once a month or zoledronate 5 mg infusion once a year (!)); (c) denosumab 60 mg subcutaneous injection once every 6 months (!); (d) oestrogen, preferably in combination with a gynaecological indication; (e) SERM (selective oestrogen receptor modulator, raloxifene); (f) strontium ranelate (oral suspension of 2 g daily), (g) calcitonin (injections of 100 IE daily) and finally (h) teriparatide (subcutaneous injections of 20 µg daily).

Arrange for *follow-up controls* and introduce the patient to an orthopaedic fracture care chain if one is available.

# Bibliography

Andersson M et al (2005) Skelett- och ledskador. Karlstad Hospital, Värmlands läns landsting, Karlstad

Bahr R, Maehlum S (eds) (2004) Idrottsskador. SISU Idrottsböcker, Stockholm

Chan KM et al (eds) (2006) Team physician manual, 2nd edn. FIMS, Hong Kong

Danielsson L, Willner S (1981) Barnortopedi och skolioser. Studentlitteratur, Lund

Ip D (2005) Orthopedic principles – a resident's guide. Springer, Berlin

Iversen L, Swiontkowski M (1995) Manual of acute orthopaedic therapeutics. Little, Brown and Company, Boston

Karlsson J (1998) Fotens sjukdomar och skador. Astra Läkemedel, Södertälje

Kasser JR (ed) (1996) Orthopaedic knowledge update 5. American Academy of Orthopaedic Surgeons, Rosemont

Kjaer M et al (eds) (2003) Textbook of sports medicine. Blackwell, Oxford

Lennquist S (2002) Katastrofmedicin. Liber, Stockholm

Lindgren U, Svensson O (2001) Ortopedi. Liber, Stockholm

Lund B (2004) Skadebogen. Forlaget IBL, Silkeborg

Lundborg G (1988) Handkirurgi – en introduktion. Studentlitteratur, Lund

Montgomery F, Lidström J (2003) Fotkirurgi. Liber, Stockholm

Netter FH (1987) Musculoskeletal system part I. CIBA Collection, Summit

Önnerfelt J, Önnerfelt R (2003) Akut ortopedi. Studentlitteratur, Lund

Read M (2000) A practical guide to sports injuries. Butterworth-Heinemann, Oxford

Snider R (ed) (1999) Essentials of musculoskeletal care. American Academy of Orthopaedic Surgeons, Rosemont

Sölveborn S-A (2004) Boken om stretching, 19th edn. SölveBok, Ystad

Sölveborn S-A (2011) Myterna inom idrott, skador och rörelseapparaten, 5th edn. SölveBok, Ystad

Sponseller PD (ed) (2001) The 5-minute orthopaedic consult. Lippincott Williams & Wilkins, Philadelphia/Baltimore

Westlin N (1992) Stora fotboken. Liber, Stockholm

S.-A. Sölveborn, *Emergency Orthopedics*,                                               243
DOI 10.1007/978-3-642-41854-9, © Springer-Verlag Berlin Heidelberg 2014

# Index

## A

Abductor pollicis longus (APL) tendons, 209
AC. *See* Acromioclavicular (AC) dislocation
Acetabular fracture, 113
Achilles insertalgia, 29
Achilles paratendinosis, 48
Achilles tendalgia
  diagnosis, 59
  treatment, 60
Achilles tendon rupture
  diagnosis
    difficulties, 52
    plantar flexion, 52–53
    sudden pain, 52
    swelling, 53
    Thompson sign/Simmonds sign, 53, 54
    ultrasound/MRI, 53
    white collar professions, 52
  surgical and nonsurgical treatment, 54
Acromioclavicular (AC) dislocation
  acromioclavicular joint with concomitant
    ruptured, 155
  diagnosis, 155
  treatment, 155
Acute calcific tendinitis
  diagnosis, 167
  puncture into, 167, 168
  treatment, 167
Acute compartment syndrome, 57
Acute lumbar pain
  difficulties, 123
  multifactorial causes, 123
  radiographs, 123
  and sacral back region, 123
  SLR test, 123, 124
  treatment, 123–124
Adductor longus insertalgia/tear, 101

AMBRII. *See* Atraumatic, multidirectional,
    bilateral, rehabilitation, inferior
    capsule, interval closure (AMBRII)
Ankle distortion
  diagnosis, 39–40
  treatment, 40
Ankle fracture. *See* Ankle injuries
Ankle injuries
  achilles tendon rupture, 42
  distortion, 39–40
  fibular tendon dislocation (*see* Fibular
    tendon dislocation)
  fracture
    in children, 41–42
    diagnosis, 41
    dislocation, 40
    Pilon, 42
    treatment, 41
  measures, 39
  swelling, 38
Ankle osteoarthrosis, 48
Ankle pain
  achilles paratendinosis, 48
  achilles tendalgia, 48
  back pain, 48
  loose body joint, 47
  osteochondral defect, 47
  osteochondrosis (dissecans) tali, 45–47
  osteoarthritis, 48
  posterior tibial tendon rupture/tendalgia
    (*see* Posterior tibial tendon rupture/
    tendalgia)
  posttraumatic synovial impingement, 45
  subdislocating fibular (peroneal) tendon, 47
Ankle puncture, injections, 237
Ankylosing spondylitis
  inflammatory disease, 130